Diagnosis of Lameness in Dogs

Diagnosis of Lameness in Dogs

Edited by

Kei Hayashi, DVM, PhD, DACVS
College of Veterinary Medicine
Cornell University
Ithaca, NY, USA

WILEY Blackwell

Registered Office
John Wiley & Sons, Inc., 111 River Street, Hoboken, NJ 07030, USA

For details of our global editorial offices, customer services, and more information about Wiley products visit us at www.wiley.com.

Wiley also publishes its books in a variety of electronic formats and by print-on-demand. Some content that appears in standard print versions of this book may not be available in other formats.

Library of Congress Cataloging-in-Publication Data applied for:

ISBN 9781118443880 (paperback), LCCN 2022053745

Cover Design: Wiley
Cover Images: Courtesy of Kei Hayashi

Set in 9.5/12.5pt STIXTwoText by Straive, Chennai, India

SKY10043962_030623

Contents

Dedication

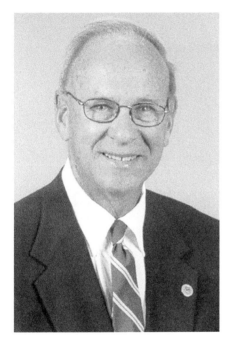

Rudolf "Tass" Dueland (1933–2018)   **Eb Rosin (1942–1999)**

I would like to dedicate this book to the following people: Drs. Tass Dueland, Eb Rosin, Mark Markel, Paul Manley, Kenneth Johnson, Gretchen Flo, Charlie DeCamp, Curtis Probst, Kathy Linn, John McAnulty, and Jay Harvey. These people dedicated their lives to teaching. We would also like to dedicate this book to all our patients.

List of Contributors

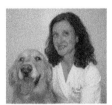

Kimberly A. Agnello, DVM, MS, Dipl. ACVS-SA, DACVSMR
Associate Professor of Small Animal Surgery
Department of Clinical Studies &
Advanced Medicine
University of Pennsylvania
School of Veterinary Medicine
Philadelphia, PA, USA
ACVS Founding Fellow
Minimally Invasive Surgery (Orthopedics)

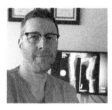

Derek B. Fox, DVM, PhD, Dipl. ACVS
Professor, Small Animal Orthopedic Surgery
Chief, Small Animal Surgical Service
Veterinary Health Center
University of Missouri
Columbia, MO, USA

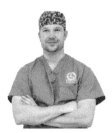

Mark C. Fuller, DVM, Dipl. ACVS-SA
Small Animal Surgeon
Fuller Animal Specialty Hospital
Calgary, AB, Canada

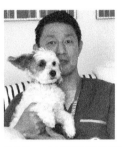

Kei Hayashi, DVM, PhD, Dipl. ACVS
Professor, Surgery
College of Veterinary Medicine
Cornell University
Ithaca, NY, USA
Adjunct Professor, University of Wisconsin
Visiting Professor, University of Tokyo

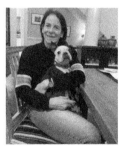

Amy S. Kapatkin, DVM, MAS, Dipl. ACVS
Professor of Orthopedic Surgery
Small Animal Orthopedic Surgery Section Chief
University of California-Davis
Davis, CA, USA
ACVS Founding Fellow, Joint Replacement Surgery

Preface

There are books on veterinary medicine that we rely on. But as we grow older and more impatient, we realize that we want a practical book with more pictures and videos than words. So, this is a book written by practicing veterinary orthopedic surgeons. We hope people short on time and patience find this book practical and that it makes it easy to understand the principles. The fundamentals are repeated over and over in different chapters. This is a real-world textbook for students, practicing veterinarians, interns, and residents.

In this book, practical methods are presented with many pictures, videos, and radiographs (sometimes supplemented by CT scan, ultrasound, MRI, and arthroscopy) of actual patients. Accurate diagnosis is a basis for all treatment options.

This textbook discusses the importance of a "problem-oriented stepwise approach."

First, identify the primary problem. Then, list differentials based on the size and age of the canine patient. However, *do not* forget to rule out nonorthopedic conditions, including medical, oncologic, and neurologic disorders.

Four practical steps are an essential part of the process for an accurate diagnosis:

- Differential list (prioritize common problems based on age and size).
- Observation (posture, sit, gait, etc.).
- Palpation (careful and thorough physical examination).
- Diagnostic imaging (mainly radiographs).

There are also links to some awesome videos, which are a crucial part of this textbook. Do check them out.

Textbooks about treatment options and surgical complications are in the works – stay tuned!

Acknowledgments

We would like to acknowledge the following people:

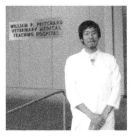

Dr. Koji Aoki for taking pictures and videos.

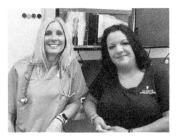

Michele Callahan and Marni McChesney, and

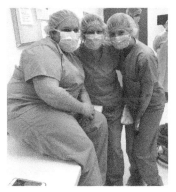

Rhea Adams, Renee Sparrow, and Kim Heath for taking care of our patients.

Geri Holzman, Carrie Lowrey, and Lisa Mailler (pictures not shown) for managing our cases.

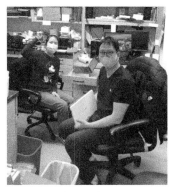

Drs. Yu Izumisawa, Sae Jong Yoo,

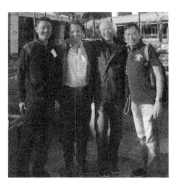

Sun Young Kim, and Po-Yen Chou for organizing data.

About the Companion Website

This book is accompanied by a companion website.

 www.wiley.com/go/hayashi/lameness

This website includes:

- Videos

Section 1

Orthopedic Examination

1

General Examination

Derek B. Fox and Amy S. Kapatkin

1.1 General Strategy

A practical, logical, and systematic approach is essential in diagnosing lameness in dogs. This chapter will describe general guidelines to achieve this goal, consisting of the following:

- *Immediate care.* Orthopedic injuries are frequently the least important injury in a heavily traumatized dog. Do not get tunnel visioned on a grossly fractured limb, but rather assess and stabilize the entire patient, concentrating on airway, breathing, and cardiovascular support, followed by a complete neurologic examination. Severely traumatized dogs with hemorrhaging wounds, unstable/open fractures, and infected joints require urgent attention.
- *Pain assessment.* Patients need to be assessed for pain. Pain medication/sedation may be administered.

10 Practical Tips for Diagnosis of Lameness in Dogs

1. Signalment Is Your Friend

The orthopedic examination can begin prior to assessment by considering the patient's signalment. The astute clinician will consider differential diagnoses based on:

- Age
- Breed
- Presenting complaint

For example, a 7-month-old German shepherd dog that presents with a 1-month history of slowly progressing weight-bearing forelimb lameness should have its elbows and shoulders examined for a variety of developmental juvenile orthopedic conditions, such as medial coronoid disease, ununited anconeal processes, shoulder or elbow osteochondrosis, and panosteitis. Obviously, there are a number of other possible differential diagnoses (see later in this chapter). While it is prudent not to become overly focused, it is also important to remember that certain breeds and ages of dogs are at risk for specific conditions.

2. Use a Systematic Approach

- *History.* The history obtained from the owner should include:
  - Duration and persistence of clinical signs.
  - Whether one limb or multiple limbs are affected.
  - If certain activities exacerbate the signs.
  - Whether the patient is a pet or a working/competing animal.

- *Observation.* Watching the animal move and observing its gait and behavior, either as it is walked or trotted by a handler or as it

Diagnosis of Lameness in Dogs, First Edition. Edited by Kei Hayashi.
© 2023 John Wiley & Sons, Inc. Published 2023 by John Wiley & Sons, Inc.
Companion website: www.wiley.com/go/hayashi/lameness

wanders around the examination room, is an important part of ascertaining the location of the lameness.

- *Physical examination*
  - Palpate the animal while it is standing.
  - Examine bilateral structures simultaneously to check for loss of symmetry, which can help detect abnormalities.
  - See if the animal can sit and rise comfortably; a variety of conditions can prohibit normal, pain-free movement during these actions.
  - Have the animal lay in lateral recumbency with the abnormal side down in order to palpate the normal limbs first.
  - Assess for range of motion, evidence of pain or instability, joint swelling, long bone sensitivity, and any other pathologic abnormalities; then repeat the process on the abnormal side.
  - Develop your own system/order of examination and repeat the same process for every patient, which ensures that nothing is forgotten or missed.

3. Understand the Goals of Orthopedic Examinations

The initial orthopedic examination serves as an extension of the physical examination, which should always be completed concomitantly. Once you lay your hands on the dog, completing an orthopedic examination is based on the detection of two fundamental findings:

- Palpating pathologic abnormalities and/or eliciting pain from the manipulation and palpation of specific anatomic structures.
- Detecting abnormalities or pain of a specific anatomic structure, which then prompts performance of additional diagnostics, such as arthrocentesis or radiography.

Many veterinarians new to orthopedic concepts fear that they are not strong enough or have hands large enough to complete certain palpation maneuvers, especially in larger animals. Remember that diagnosis of a condition is rarely reliant on a single physical finding.

For example, if you cannot adequately manipulate the stifle of a mastiff to assess the cranial cruciate ligament (CCL) for cranial drawer, you can palpate for stifle effusion, medial buttress, and pain upon flexion or extension, all of which potentially indicate a ruptured CCL.

4. Perform a Neurologic Examination

Many sources of lameness and muscle atrophy are attributable to neurologic conditions, which must be distinguished from musculoskeletal conditions as they may require more immediate attention. Examples include cervical intervertebral disk herniation (forelimb lameness) and lumbosacral disease (hindlimb lameness). The neurologic examination can be done before, after, or even during the orthopedic examination.

- Support the standing animal under the chest and pelvis during spinal palpation of the thoracic and lumbar spine, respectively.
- Assess for spinal hyperpathia by putting the head and neck through a range of motion (as long as they are not "neck guarding"), deeply palpating the thoracic and lumbar spine, and lifting the tail.
- Lift their hips and perform a lordosis examination, assessing for pain.
- Check conscious proprioception of all four limbs by knuckling the paws and examining the reaction.
- With the animal in lateral recumbency, assess the spinal reflexes, both myotactic and withdrawal.

Completing these examinations is essential and will help diagnose neurologic conditions that may be the culprit behind the lameness, atrophy, or ataxia.

5. Use Sedation for Radiographs and Palpation

For fractious or painful animals, the orthopedic examination may be very stressful or painful. Sedation will allow a more complete examination. Prior to the completion of radiographs, or any diagnostic imaging modality, the clinician should have a suspicion of which anatomic region is the source of pain and a list of potential differential diagnoses affecting the patient based on the orthopedic examination. The radiographic findings, then, should either support or refute the suspicions generated during palpation. There are numerous advantages to sedating a patient for radiographs, including:

- Alleviation of stress resulting from restraint, which can be painful.
- Prevention of movement, resulting in a higher likelihood of getting a well-positioned, accurately exposed radiograph with fewer attempts, reducing radiation exposure to everyone involved, including the patient.

Consult with an anesthesiologist for safe protocols and always monitor your patients closely while they are sedated for any signs of cardiovascular or respiratory compromise. Be ready to reverse the sedation or immediately establish an airway if needed. A safe and effective reversible cocktail used at our hospital for both dogs and cats is dexmedetomidine (5 µg/kg) and butorphanol (0.5 mg/kg). If the animal is particularly painful, you can substitute morphine for the butorphanol and, if overly fractious, the dose of the dexmedetomidine can be doubled.

6. Practice Specific Palpation Maneuvers under Sedation

Much of the orthopedic examination consists of palpating for pathologic changes, and a number of specific palpation maneuvers exist that are highly specific and sensitive to particular joints and conditions. Examples include:

- *Stifle* – palpating for cranial drawer and tibial thrust for a ruptured CCL.
- *Patella* – palpating for instability through stifle flexion and extension and internal and external rotation of the tibia.
- *Coxofemoral subluxation* – assessment for laxity via examination for Barden and Ortolani signs.

Proficiency and accuracy come from experience and these maneuvers must be practiced regularly in order to distinguish what is normal versus abnormal. A good practice is to perform them on any sedated or anesthetized patient in your hospital (especially the Ortolani examination in young dogs that are under anesthesia for ovariohysterectomy). Not only will you gain comfort and accuracy in executing the maneuvers, but you may also diagnose preclinical hip dysplasia in more than a few dogs.

7. Repeat Radiographic Positioning Identically Every Time

Reading orthopedic radiographs is often pattern recognition. For example, when reading pelvic radiographs of a dog for evidence of hip dysplasia, look for specific signs, including femoral head coverage, osteophytosis along the femoral neck, and remodeling of the femoral head. It is essential that the pelvis is positioned straight and in an identical fashion in every patient radiographed. By doing so, the clinician can avoid the distraction of trying to interpret artifacts that inevitable result from poor positioning.

Similarly, always examine your films in the same orientation. In our hospital, we have a saying that "all dogs run to the left," meaning that radiographs of all joints and long bones have the cranial view oriented to the viewer's left. This way, the eye does not become confused by viewing differently oriented joints and bones, but rather can focus on signs of pathology instead.

8. Know What Radiographic Signs of Osteoarthritis Mean

When you are taking radiographs of a painful joint, the anatomic structure responsible for the instability is frequently not seen. The perfect example is a knee that has suffered a rupture of the CCL. The torn ligament and subsequent meniscal tears are not radiographically visible despite the fact that both are potential sources of lameness. Similarly, fragmentation of the medial coronoid process may not be specifically visualized on a radiograph of a young dog with elbow dysplasia. What are noticeable in these cases, however, are the subsequent radiographic signs of secondary osteoarthritis. These include:

- Osteophytosis along the joint margin
- Joint effusion
- Subchondral sclerosis

Young and middle-aged dogs rarely get primary osteoarthritis of the major diarthrodial joints, so such changes are usually indicative of underlying pathology.

9. Don't Be Afraid of Arthrocentesis

Arthrocentesis is crucial for:

- Distinguishing arthropathies as suppurative (such as immune-mediated poly-arthropathy [IMPA] or Lyme disease) from nonsuppurative via cytologic examination.
- Obtaining synovial fluid for culture and susceptibility if septic arthritis is suspected.

Many veterinarians are afraid of "tapping" a joint for fear of doing damage to structures within it. While this is a valid concern, with a little practice and review of anatomy arthrocentesis can be a straightforward and low-risk procedure.

- Practice good aseptic technique by shaving and scrubbing the skin with an antiseptic solution, wearing sterile gloves, and using sterile needles (22- or 25-gauge depending on the patient's size) and syringes.
- Be familiar with the anatomy of the joint in question to avoid major arteries, veins, nerves, and myotendinous structures.
- Palpate for the point of maximal joint distension and direct your needle there. For highly effusive joints (which constitute a large number of cases that require arthrocentesis), the capsule is distended with fluid and the area of greatest distension is frequently where the aforementioned structures you wish to avoid are not present. For joints that are less effusive, distension (the bulge) can be created by pressing on the opposite side of the joint.

- Once the needle is in, it may be redirected slightly or its depth altered if you are unable to withdraw fluid easily.
- Withdraw the needle if your sample becomes tinged with blood. The sample is still usable, but limiting blood contamination makes it easier to evaluate.

10. Pursue Advice and Continuing Education

Becoming proficient in orthopedics isn't just mastering fracture repair or arthroscopy. Rather, making early and accurate diagnoses and instituting appropriate medical management of orthopedic conditions are paramount to the long-term prognosis of the patient, especially if surgery is ultimately required. When in doubt, get help, either by calling for advice from a surgeon who specializes in orthopedic surgery or attending seminars or any number of the continuing education opportunities available.

1.2 Chief Complaint and History

The patient's general health should be assured before focusing on the orthopedic complaint. In addition to the chief complaint(s), the patient's relevant medical history, a history of recent trauma, living environment (such as indoor/outdoor, other animals in a household), the intended use of the patient (e.g., family pet, breeding, showing, racing, or hunting dog), and expectation/treatment goals should be obtained before performing a physical examination.

History

Specific historical information is useful for categorizing orthopedic problems to rule out. This information includes:

- Owner identification of limb(s) involved (chief complaint).
- Breed (size), age, sex.
- Onset, potential trauma.
- Chronological progression of the problem.
- Efficacy of treatments tried.

- Variability with weather, time of the day (morning vs. evening), exercise, and arising from recumbency.

Other features, such as fever, inappetence, lethargy, and weight loss, may indicate some systemic problem.

Certain historical facts and deviation from the "normal" presentation of particular orthopedic conditions alert the clinician to investigate further by asking appropriate questions or performing additional tests or procedures. For example:

- Chronic luxating patella usually does not suddenly cause a lameness, and CCL rupture may have become the more recent problem.
- A 10-year-old dog that falls down and sustains a fractured radius and ulna should be carefully scrutinized for pathologic fracture (neoplasia).
- Chronic osteoarthritic conditions usually do not cause severe pain. In older animals with severe progressive pain, neoplasia must always be considered.
- With pelvic fractures, trauma to the chest, abdomen, or spine often occurs.

Urgent Conditions

Particularly for trauma patients, serious systemic and neurologic problems must be ruled out before focusing on orthopedic complaint.

Answers to specific questions help assess concurrent problems. For example:

- A good appetite probably does not occur with significant internal injuries.
- "Urinating" or dribbling small amounts of urine does *not* mean the bladder is intact.
- Voluntary leg movement usually means serious thoracolumbar spinal injury has not occurred.

1.3 Rule-Outs: Systemic (Medical) Conditions and Neurologic Disorders

Once the patient is determined to be stable, nonorthopedic causes of lameness must be ruled out before focusing on orthopedic conditions (see Table 1.1).

Systemic Conditions

Generalized weakness due to systemic illness may mimic a lameness. These medical conditions, including malnutrition and endocrinopathy, must be suspected by veterinarian's clinical judgment. Severe skin problems (such as interdigital dermatitis) in the toe area may also cause lameness.

Table 1.1 Medical and neurologic rule-outs in lameness.

Category	Common condition	Example
Medical	Immune-mediated	Immune-mediated poly-arthropathy
	Endocrinopathy	Cushing, diabetes
	Infectious	Lyme disease
Neurologic	Congenital/degenerative	Lumbosacral disease
	Disc disease	T3-L3 myelopathy
		Cervical myelopathy
	Degenerative	Degenerative myelopathy

Poly-arthropathy

IPMA and some infectious diseases (such as Lyme disease) can cause multiple joint swelling and pain. Patients with these conditions may present to the hospital with a chief complaint of lameness. The patients may also show lethargy and fever. These medical conditions must be suspected by the veterinarian's clinical judgment.

Neurologic Conditions

Neurologic conditions must be distinguished from orthopedic conditions, as they may require more immediate attention. Examples include cervical intervertebral disk herniation (forelimb lameness) and lumbosacral disease (hindlimb lameness). Conditions such as disc disease, neuromuscular disorders, and degenerative myelopathy typically show neurologic signs, which should be distinguished from lameness (Dewey & da Costa 2015).

1.4 Differential Diagnosis

Common causes of lameness should be listed, mainly based on the size and age of the patient (Tables 1.2–1.4). It must be noted that lameness can be a result of a combination of multiple conditions. For example:

- CCL rupture (cruciate disease) and hip osteoarthritis (OA).
- Hip OA and lumbosacral disease.
- Medial patellar luxation and cruciate disease.

Forelimb Lameness in Small-Breed/ Skeletally Immature Dogs

General/Multiple
- Trauma – fracture, luxation.
- Atlantoaxial luxation.
- Epiphyseal dysplasia, "Swimmers."

Shoulder Region
- Congenital luxation and glenoid hypoplasia.

Elbow Region
- Congenital luxation.
- Subluxation caused by premature physeal closure or breed (chondrodystrophic) predisposition (angular limb deformity [ALD]).
- Fracture from incomplete ossification of the humeral condyle (also mature dogs and all sizes).

Carpal Region
- Subluxation caused by premature physeal closure (ALD).
- Carpal laxity

Forelimb Lameness in Small-Breed/ Skeletally Mature Dogs

General/Multiple
- Trauma – fracture, luxation, muscle and nerve injuries.
- Cervical lesion – disk, tumor.
- Brachial plexus tumor.
- Hypertrophic osteopathy (HO).

Shoulder Region
- Degenerative joint disease (DJD)/OA.
- Recurrent medial luxation, nontraumatic.

Elbow Region
- DJD/OA.
- Subluxation caused by physeal injury (ALD).

Carpal Region
- DJD/OA.
- Inflammatory joint disease (IMPA) and erosive arthropathy.
- Subluxation caused by prior physeal injury (ALD).

Forelimb Lameness in Large-Breed/ Skeletally Immature Dogs

General/Multiple
- Trauma – fracture, luxation.
- Panosteitis (PO).
- Hypertrophic osteodystrophy (HOD).
- Cervical lesion, vertebral instability.

Table 1.2   General/multiple limb conditions (nonorthopedic conditions in italics).

	Small-breed Growing	Small-breed Mature	Large-breed Growing	Large-breed Mature
Common	*Atlantoaxial luxation*	*IMPA* *Cervical lesion* *Infectious (Lyme)*	*Panostitis* *Cervical lesion*	*Cervical lesion* *IMPA* *Infectious (Lyme)*
Rare	"Swimmers"	HO	HOD	HO

HO, hypertrophic osteopathy; HOD, hypertrophic osteodystrophy; IMPA, immune-mediated poly-arthropathy.

Table 1.3   Thoracic limb conditions (nonorthopedic conditions in italics).

	Small-breed Growing	Small-breed Mature	Large-breed Growing	Large-breed Mature
Common	Radius/ulna fracture Condylar fracture Congenital luxation ALD	Radius/ulna fracture Condylar fracture Shoulder luxation *Cervical lesion*	Elbow dysplasia Panostitis Shoulder OCD ALD	*Neoplasia* *Cervical lesion* Elbow OA Shoulder tendinopathy Carpal hyperextension
Rare	Carpal laxity Septic arthritis Physitis	HO Septic arthritis Osteomyelitis *Neoplasia*	HOD Congenital luxation Septic arthritis Physitis	HO Septic arthritis Osteomyelitis Sesamoid disease

ALD, angular limb deformity; HO, hypertrophic osteopathy; HOD, hypertrophic osteodystrophy; OA, osteoarthritis; OCD, osteochondritis dissecans.

Table 1.4   Pelvic limb conditions (nonorthopedic conditions in italics).

	Small-breed Growing	Small-breed Mature	Large-breed Growing	Large-breed Mature
Common	Patellar luxation Avascular necrosis Physeal fractures	Cruciate disease Hip luxation Patellar luxation Hip OA	Hip dysplasia Panostitis Tarsal/stifle OCD Patellar luxation Physeal fractures	*Neoplasia* *LS disease* Cruciate disease Hip OA Tendinopathy
Rare	Hip dysplasia Septic arthritis Physitis *Spinal deformities* Tibial deformity	*Neoplasia* *LS disease* HO Septic arthritis Osteomyelitis	HOD Osgood–Schlatter Septic arthritis Osteomyelitis Avulsion fractures	HO Septic arthritis Osteomyelitis SDF dislocation

HO, hypertrophic osteopathy; HOD, hypertrophic osteodystrophy; LS, lumbosacral; OA, osteoarthritis; OCD, osteochondritis dissecans; SDF, superficial digital flexor.

Shoulder Region
- Osteochondritis dissecans (OCD) of humeral head.
- Congenital luxation and glenoid hypoplasia.

Elbow Region
- Fragmentation of medial coronoid process (FCP)/medial coronoid disease (MCD) (elbow dysplasia).
- OCD of medial trochlear ridge (elbow dysplasia).
- Ununited anconeal process (UAP) (elbow dysplasia).
- Enthesopathy, tendinopathy, avulsion, and calcification of the flexor tendons of the medial epicondyle or ununited medial epicondyle (UME).
- Subluxation caused by premature physeal closure and ALD.
- Incongruity.
- Congenital luxation.

Carpal Region
- Subluxation/valgus or varus deformity caused by premature physeal closure (ALD).
- Valgus deformity caused by retained cartilage cores (RCC) in the ulna, or ALD.

Forelimb Lameness in Large-Breed/Skeletally Mature Dogs

General/Multiple
- Trauma – fracture, luxation, muscle and nerve injuries.
- Cervical lesion – disk, tumor, vertebral instability.
- Brachial plexus tumor.
- Bone, cartilage, or synovial tumor.
- HO.

Shoulder Region
- Secondary OA, synovitis, and tendinitis to OCD of humeral head.
- DJD/OA, primary or secondary.
- Contracture of infraspinatus muscle.
- Tenosynovitis of biceps brachii tendon.
- Calcification of supraspinatus muscle.
- Luxation/instability.

Elbow Region
- DJD/OA secondary to elbow dysplasia.
- Traumatic (jump-down) FCP.
- Enthesopathy or calcification of the flexor tendons.
- Subluxation caused by prior physeal injury or breed (chondrodystrophic) predisposition (ALD).
- Subluxation caused by premature physeal closure (ALD).

Carpal Region
- Ligamentous instability/hyperextension.
- Subluxation caused by premature physeal closure (ALD).
- DJD/OA.
- Inflammatory joint disease, with (erosive arthropathy) or without instability (IMPA).

Paw Region
- Fragmentation of the sesamoids.

Pelvic Limb Lameness in Small-Breed/Skeletally Immature Dogs

General/Multiple
- Trauma – fracture, luxation.
- Epiphyseal dysplasia, "Swimmers."

Hip Region
- Avascular necrosis (Legg–Calve–Perthes).
- Hip dysplasia, subluxation.
- Hip luxation.

Stifle Region
- Luxating patella complex.

Tarsal Region
- Tibial deformity (Miniature Dachshund).

Pelvic Limb Lameness in Small-Breed/Skeletally Mature Dogs

General/Multiple
- Trauma – fracture, luxation, muscle and nerve injuries.
- T3–L3 myelopathy.

- Lumbosacral disease (cauda equina syndrome).
- Bone, cartilage, or synovial tumor.
- HO.

Hip Region
- DJD/OA.
- Hip luxation.

Stifle Region
- Luxating patella complex.
- Cruciate/meniscal syndrome (cruciate disease).

Tarsal Region
- Achilles' tendon injury/inflammation.
- Superficial digital flexor (SDF) tendon dislocations (Toy Poodles).
- Inflammatory joint disease, with (erosive arthropathy) or without instability (IMPA).

Pelvic Limb Lameness in Large-Breed/ Skeletally Immature Dogs

General/Multiple
- Trauma – fracture, luxation.
- PO.
- HOD.
- Congenital spinal deformity.

Hip Region
- Hip dysplasia.
- Capital physeal fracture.

Stifle Region
- OCD of lateral condyle.
- Luxating patella complex.
- Avulsion of long digital extensor or cruciate ligaments.
- Genu valgum.

Tarsal Region
- Valgus or varus deformity caused by premature physeal closure.

Pelvic Limb Lameness in Large-Breed/ Skeletally Mature Dogs

General/Multiple
- Trauma – fracture, luxation, muscle and nerve injuries.
- T3–L3 myelopathy.
- Lumbosacral disease (cauda equina syndrome).
- Bone, cartilage, or synovial tumor.
- HO.

Hip Region
- DJD/OA, primary or secondary.
- Iliopsoas tendinitis.
- Lumbosacral disease (cauda equina syndrome).

Stifle Region
- Cruciate/meniscal syndrome (cruciate disease).
- Bone or synovial tumor.

Tarsal Region
- Achilles tendon injury/inflammation.
- SDF tendon dislocations (Collies and Shelties).
- DJD/OA secondary to OCD.
- Inflammatory joint disease, with (erosive arthropathy) or without instability (IMPA).

1.5 Orthopedic Examination Form

Observation of stance, sit, and gait, neurologic examination, and systematic palpation of specific anatomic structures will generate a short list of presumptive diagnoses in most orthopedic conditions (Tables 1.5 and 1.6).

The presumptive diagnoses based on the orthopedic examination should be followed up with diagnostic imaging (radiography, ultrasonography, or other imaging) to confirm the diagnosis and provide clients with treatment options and prognoses.

Table 1.5 Example of an orthopedic examination form (comprehensive version).

Date: _____   ID: _____   Name: _____

Examiner: _____   Breed: _____

_____   Age: _____   DOB: _____

BW: _____   BCS: __/9__   Sex: F/SF/M/NM

CC: _____

History: _____

Lameness: Acute / Chronic / Intermittent / Progressive / Other: _____

Pattern: Constant / When Rising / Morning / After Exercise / After Rest / Other: _____

Medication: _____

General Statue: Normal / Depressed / Non-Ambulatory / Other: _____

Appetite Y / N; Vomit Y / N; Diarrhea Y / N; Fever Y / N; Other: _____

Attitude: Cooperative / Anxious / Stressed / Aggressive / Tense / Relaxed / Other: _____

√ Check all that apply:

Posture	None (Normal)	Thoracic		Pelvic		Note
		Left	Right	Left	Right	
Knuckling						
Limb Lifting						
Obvious Swelling						
Deformity						
Carpus/Hock Down						
Positive Sit Test						

Gait	None (Normal)	Walk				Trot			
		Thoracic		Pelvic		Thoracic		Pelvic	
		Left	Right	Left	Right	Left	Right	Left	Right
Knuckling									
Short Stride									
↓ Weight Bearing									
Head Bob									
Hip Hike									
Hip Swing									
Skip/Kick									

Lameness Score	0: None	1: Intermittent	2: Mild (Weight Bearing)	3: Moderate (Toe-Touching)	4: Severe (Non-Weight Bearing)

	Thoracic: Left Right	Pelvic: Left Right
Walk	_____ _____	_____ _____
Trot	_____ _____	_____ _____

Note (Gait in Circle, or Stairs): _____

Overall Gait Description: _____

(Continued)

Table 1.5 (Continued)

√ Check that applies:

Quick Standing Neuro Exam	None (Normal)		Note
CP Deficits: Thoracic Limb		Left Right	
CP Deficits: Pelvic Limb		Left Right	
Pain: Neck Palpation			
Pain: Neck Flexion/Extension			
Thoracolumbar Pain			
Lumbosacral Pain			
Tail Elevation Pain			

Standing Exam Thoracic Limb	None (Normal)	Thoracic		Note
		Left	Right	
Scapular Displacement				
Scapular Muscle Atrophy				
Shoulder Flexion Pain				
Shoulder Extension Pain				
Proximal Humeral Pain				
Elbow Swelling/Effusion				
Pain: Medial Coronoid Region				
Elbow Flexion Pain				
Elbow Extension Pain				
Proximal Ulnar Pain				
Distal Radial Pain				
Carpal Swelling				

Standing Exam Pelvic Limb	None (Normal)	Pelvic		Note
		Left	Right	
Displaced Greater Trochanter				
Biceps Muscle Atrophy				
Hip Extension Pain				
Mid-Thigh Muscle Atrophy				
Caudal Thigh Pain/Fibrosis				
Stifle Swelling				
Stifle Effusion				
Pain on Medial Stifle				
Pain on Stifle Extension				
Tibial Thrust				
Medial Patellar Luxation				
Lateral Patellar Luxation				
Femoral Bone Pain				
Tibial Bone Pain				
Calcaneal Tendon Swelling				
Tarsal Swelling/Effusion				

(Continued)

Table 1.5 (Continued)

Recumbent Exam Thoracic Limb	None (Normal)	Thoracic		Note
		Left	Right	
↓Withdraw Reflex				
Nail/Pad/Digit Pain/Swelling				
Metacarpal Pain				
Carpal Swelling/Effusion				
Carpal Flexion/Extension Pain/↓ROM				
Carpal Instability				
Radial/Ulna Bone Pain				
Elbow Swelling/Effusion				
Elbow Flexion/Extension Pain/↓ROM				
Elbow Rotational Instability/Pain				
Pain: Medial Coronoid Region				
Humeral Bone Pain				
Shoulder Flexion/Extension Pain				
Shoulder Flexion/Elbow Extension Pain				
Shoulder Abduction Instability/Pain				
Pain: Axillary Region				
Scapular Bone Pain				

Recumbent Exam Pelvic Limb	None (Normal)	Pelvic		Note
		Left	Right	
↓Withdraw Reflex				
Nail/Pad/Digit Pain/Swelling				
Metatarsal Pain				
Tarsal Swelling/Effusion				
Tarsal Flexion/Extension Pain				
Tarsal Instability				
Calcaneal Tendon Swelling/Pain				
Superficial Digital Flexor Dislocation				
Tibial/Fibular bone Pain				
↓Patellar Reflex				
Stifle Swelling				
Stifle Flexion/Extension Pain/↓ROM				
Medial/Lateral Patellar Luxation				
Tibial Thrust/Cranial Drawer				
Stifle Collateral Instability				
Femoral Bone Pain				
Caudal Thigh Muscle Pain				
Hip Extension/Abduction Pain				
Iliopsoas/Pectineus Pain				
Hip Instability/Luxation				
Lumbosacral/Lordosis Pain				

Table 1.6 Example of an orthopedic examination form (simple version).

Date: _____ ID: _____ Name: _____

Examiner: _____ Breed: _____

_____ Age: _____ DOB: _____

BW: _____ BCS: _____ /9 Sex: F/SF/M/NM

CC: _____

History: _____

Lameness: Acute / Chronic / Intermittent / Progressive / Other: _____

Pattern: Constant / When Rising / Morning / After Exercise / After Rest / Other: _____

Medication: _____

Ambulatory Exam:

Lameness Score	0: None	1: Intermittent	2: Mild (Weight Bearing)	3: Moderate (Toe-Touching)	4: Severe (Non-Weight Bearing)

Lameness Score at Walk: _____ Limb 1(Circle): LF/RF/LH/RH   Note: _____

(Lameness Score at Walk: _____ Limb 2(Circle): LF/RF/LH/RH   Note: _____)

Lameness Score at Trot: _____ Limb 1(Circle): LF/RF/LH/RH   Note: _____

(Lameness Score at Trot: _____ Limb 2(Circle): LF/RF/LH/RH   Note: _____)

Note (Gait in Circle, or Stairs): _____

Overall Gait Description: _____

Standing Exam:

CP Deficits: No   Yes (Location): _____

Spinal Pain: No   Yes (Location): _____

Deformity: No   Yes (Location): _____

Less Weight Bearing: No   Yes (Location): _____

Muscle Asymmetry: No   Yes (Location): _____

Joint Effusion: No   Yes (Location): _____

Joint Hyperflexion: No   Yes (Location): _____

Medial Coronoid Pain: No   Yes (Circle):   LF   RF   Both

Stifle Pain: No   Yes (Circle):   LH   RH   Both

Medial Buttress: No   Yes (Circle):   LH   RH   Both

Patella Luxation: No   Yes (Direction and Grade): Med   Lat   1   2   3   4

(Continued)

Table 1.6 (Continued)

Recumbent Neuro Exam:

Withdraw Reflex:	Normal	Delayed (Circle)	LF RF LH RH
Patellar Reflex:	Normal	Absent (Circle)	LH RH
		Hyper (Circle)	LH RH

Recumbent Exam: (Note abnormal findings)

Abnormality	S: Swelling	P: Pain on Palpation	D: Decreased ROM	F/E: Pain on Full Flexion/Extension	I: Instability	C: Crepitation

Front — **Left** — **Right**

Front	Left	Right
Paw	_____	_____
Carpus	_____	_____
Radius/Ulna	_____	_____
Elbow	_____	_____
Humerus	_____	_____

Shoulder (Abduction Test, Biceps Test, Biceps Palpation, Axillary Region, Scapula)

Hind — **Left** — **Right**

Hind	Left	Right
Paw	_____	_____
Tarsus (Calcaneal Tendon)	_____	_____
Tibia/Fibula	_____	_____
Stifle	_____	_____
Patella Luxation	Medial/Lateral Grade 1 2 3 4	Medial/Lateral Grade 1 2 3 4
Meniscal Click	Mil Severe	Mild Severe
Thrust Test	Mild Severe Uncertain	Mild Severe Uncertain
Drawer Test	Mild Severe Uncertain	Mild Severe Uncertain
Femur	_____	_____

Hip (Abduction, Dorsal Luxation Test, Subluxation test)

Lumbosacral (Compression, Lordosis Test) _____

Differential Diagnosis: _____

BCS, body condition score; BW, body weight; CP, conscious proprioception; LF, left front; LH, left hind; RF, right front; RH, right hind; ROM, range of motion.

Reference

Dewey, C.W., & da Costa, R.C. (2015). *Practical Guide to Canine and Feline Neurology*, 3rd ed. Chichester: Wiley-Blackwell.

2

Orthopedic Observation

Amy S. Kapatkin

2.1 Distant Observation

Distant observation should include evaluation of:

- General/body conformation
- Abnormal stance/posture
- Decreased weight bearing
- Muscle asymmetry and atrophy
- Asymmetrical joint or soft tissue swellings
- Limb, joint, and digit alignment
- Gross joint laxity

General/Body Conformation

General Observation
See Figures 2.1 and 2.2.

Body Conformation
See Figure 2.3.

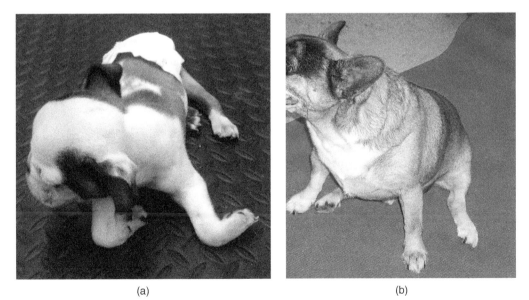

(a)   (b)

Figure 2.1 (a, b) Inability to rise may be seen with severe congenital conditions in puppies such as hydrocephalus (not orthopedic), or myelopathy in mature dogs (not orthopedic).

Diagnosis of Lameness in Dogs, First Edition. Edited by Kei Hayashi.
© 2023 John Wiley & Sons, Inc. Published 2023 by John Wiley & Sons, Inc.
Companion website: www.wiley.com/go/hayashi/lameness

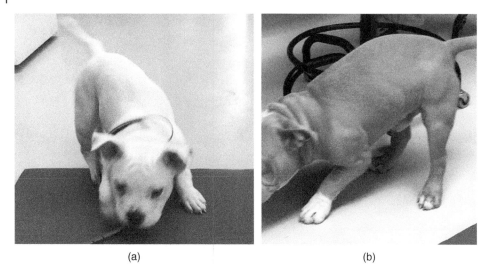

(a) (b)

Figure 2.2 (a, b) Inability to rise may be seen in puppies with congenital conditions such as congenital elbow luxation.

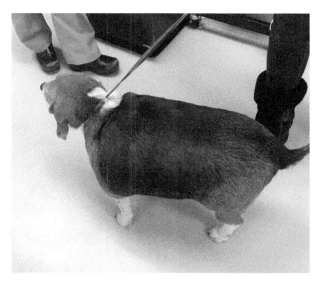

Figure 2.3 Obesity and body condition score must be noted in the medical record. Monitoring the body condition score is essential in the management of osteoarthritis (OA).

Abnormal Stance/Posture Suggestive of Neurologic Disorders

See Figures 2.4–2.6.

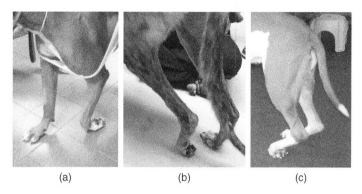

(a) (b) (c)

Figure 2.4 (a–c) "Knuckling" is often suggestive of neurologic disorders such as brachial plexus avulsion and sciatic neuropathy (not orthopedic).

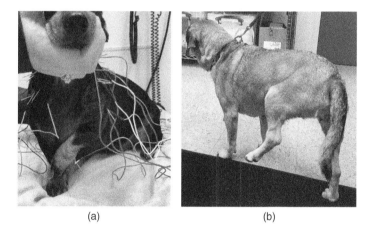

(a) (b)

Figure 2.5 (a, b) "Holding up a leg" or "root signature" is often suggestive of neurologic disorders such as lateralized disc herniation or foraminal stenosis (not orthopedic). Courtesy of Drs. Curtis Dewey and Evelyn Galban.

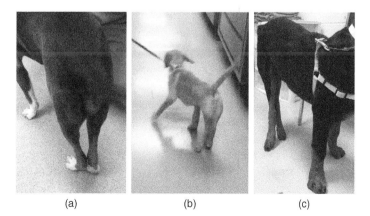

(a) (b) (c)

Figure 2.6 (a–c) Severely narrow stance or abnormal posture with bilateral stifle hyperextension may indicate severe congenital neuromuscular disorders.

Decreased Weight Bearing

See Figures 2.7–2.10.

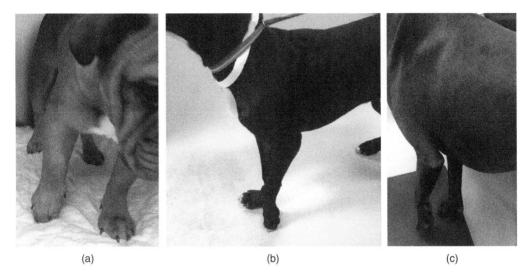

(a)   (b)   (c)

Figure 2.7 (a–c) Non-weight-bearing stance of the thoracic limb may indicate injuries to the elbow (such as elbow fracture or luxation) or injuries to the distal limb (such as pad laceration).

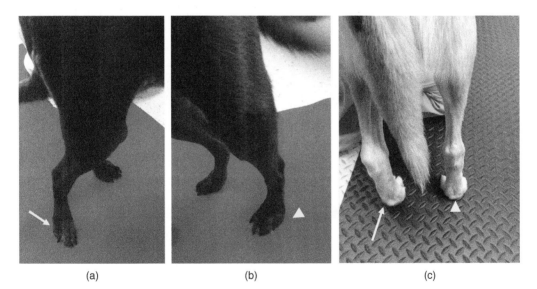

(a)   (b)   (c)

Figure 2.8 (a–c) Degree of weight bearing should be carefully observed. Partial weight-bearing "offloading" stance (arrows) – compared to the other side (arrowheads) – can be seen with orthopedic conditions such as cruciate disease.

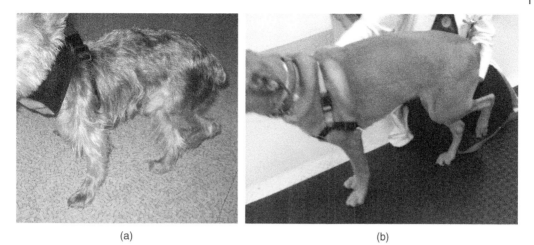

(a)   (b)

Figure 2.9 (a, b) Degree of weight bearing should be carefully observed. Completely non-weight-bearing "holding up the leg high" stance can be neurologic from nerve root pain ("root signature," see Figure 2.5) or can be seen with orthopedic conditions such as medial patellar luxation or pad laceration.

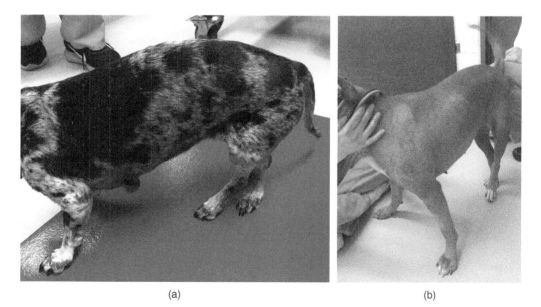

(a)   (b)

Figure 2.10 (a, b) Degree of weight bearing should be carefully observed. Non-weight-bearing "holding up" stance with external rotation and adduction of the limb can be seen with orthopedic conditions such as cranio-dorsal hip luxation.

Muscle Asymmetry and Atrophy

See Figure 2.11.

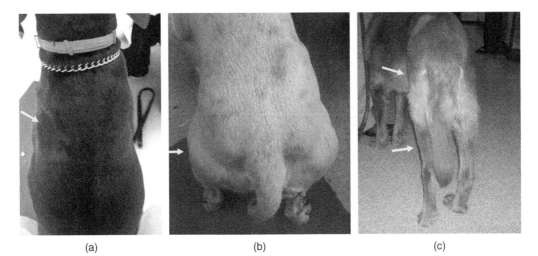

(a) (b) (c)

Figure 2.11 Obvious muscle asymmetry and atrophy should be carefully observed. (a) Thoracic limb muscle atrophy around the scapula (arrow) due to biceps tendon partial rupture. (b) Pelvic limb muscle atrophy (arrow) around the biceps femoris muscle due to hip OA. (c) Pelvic limb muscle atrophy affecting entire limb (arrows) due to combination of lateral patellar luxation and hip dysplasia.

Swelling

See Figures 2.12–2.17.

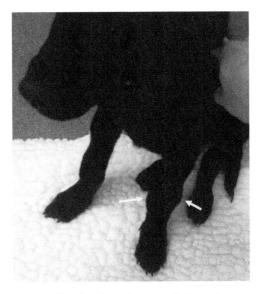

Figure 2.12 Swelling of thoracic limb can be seen in stance or sit. Bilateral swelling near carpal joints (arrows) due to hypertrophic osteodystrophy (HOD) in a puppy.

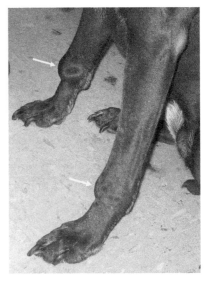

Figure 2.13 Joint swelling of thoracic limb can be seen in stance or sit. Bilateral carpal effusion (arrows) due to systemic conditions such as immune-mediated poly-arthropathy (IMPA) and Lyme disease.

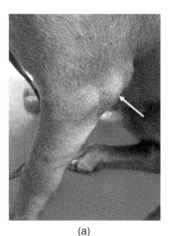

(a)

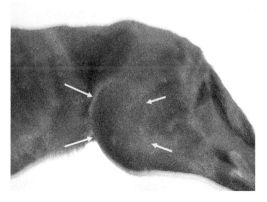

(b)

Figure 2.14 (a, b) Joint swelling of thoracic limb can be seen in stance or sit. Elbow effusion (arrow) due to severe elbow dysplasia.

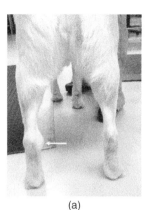

(a)

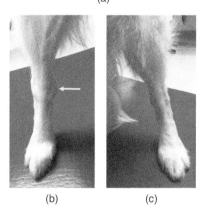

(b)   (c)

Figure 2.16 (a–c) Unilateral joint swelling of medial aspect of the tarsal joint (arrow) can be seen in weight-bearing stance from either cranial or caudal views. This is commonly seen in unilateral tarsal osteochondritis dissecans (OCD).

Figure 2.15 Severe soft tissue swelling around the stifle (arrows) may indicate neoplasia or severe infection.

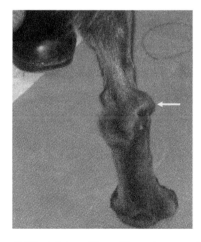

Figure 2.17 Joint swelling of lateral aspect of the tarsal joint (arrow) can be seen in weight-bearing stance with an orthopedic condition such as chronic tarsal OA.

Limb Alignment: Antebrachial Angular Limb Deformity

See Figure 2.18.

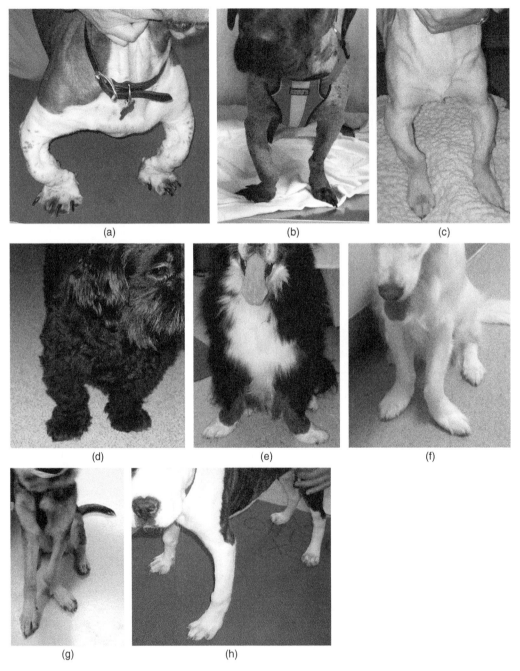

(a)

(b)

(c)

(d)

(e)

(f)

(g)

(h)

Figure 2.18 (a–h) Antebrachial angular limb deformity (ALD) caused by prior physeal injury, premature physeal closure, or breed (chondrodystrophic) predisposition can be seen in growing dogs bilaterally or unilaterally.

Limb Alignment: Hind Limb Conformation

See Figures 2.19–2.26.

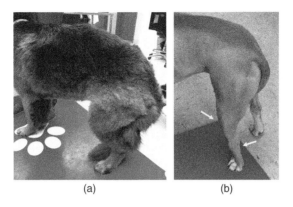

(a)   (b)

Figure 2.19 (a) "Low hind end" posture with flexed joints may be normal in some breeds such as German Shepherd, but may indicate abnormalities such as lumbosacral disease, transitional vertebrae, or bilateral stifle pain. (b) "Straight limb" with extended joints (arrows) may be normal in some breeds such as Pitbull, but is commonly associated with hip pain or cruciate disease.

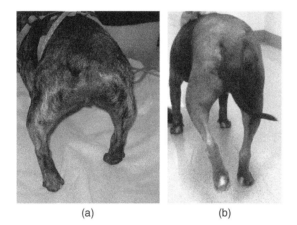

(a)   (b)

Figure 2.20 (a, b) "Bowed leg" (genu varum) posture may be normal in some breeds such as French Bulldog, but may be associated with medial patellar luxation.

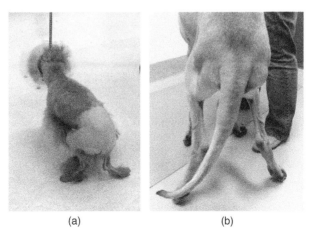

(a)   (b)

Figure 2.21 (a, b) "Knocked knee" (genu valgum) posture may be associated with severe (grade 4) lateral patellar luxation in toy or giant breed dogs.

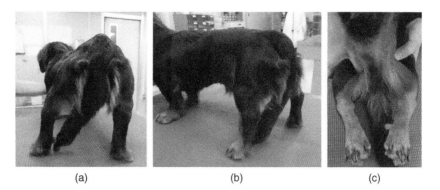

(a)   (b)   (c)

Figure 2.22 (a–c) "Pes varus" is most commonly seen in Dachshunds and may be bilateral and cause gait abnormality. Courtesy of Dr. Madoka Amano.

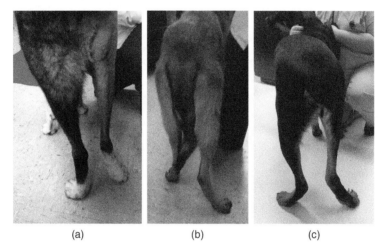

(a)   (b)   (c)

Figure 2.23 (a–c) "External rotation of the pes" and tibia valga may be associated with tibial deformity, lateral patellar luxation, or tarsal deformity.

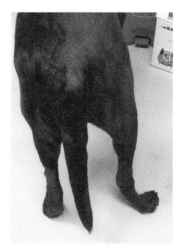

Figure 2.24 "External rotation of the pes" and tibia valga may be associated with a surgical complication of tibial fracture repaired with a poor fracture reduction from "too straight" plate or a "too big" intramedullary pin.

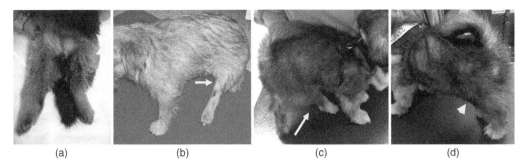

(a)　　　　　(b)　　　　　(c)　　　　　(d)

Figure 2.25　(a–d) Unilateral stifle hyperextension (genu recurvatum; arrows) may be associated with quadriceps contracture ("tie down") or a congenital condition (arrowheads: normal side).

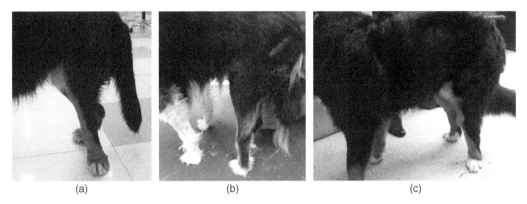

(a)　　　　　(b)　　　　　(c)

Figure 2.26　(a–c) Tarsal hyperextension is often associated with severe hip pain, but the exact mechanism of this abnormal stance is not fully understood.

Limb Alignment: Digit

See Figure 2.27.

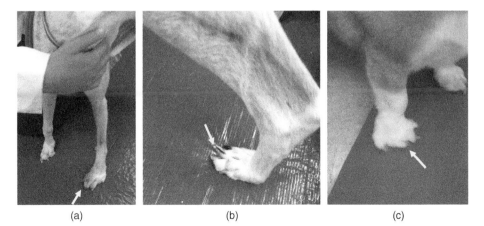

(a)　　　　　(b)　　　　　(c)

Figure 2.27　(a–c) Digital deviation (arrows) is often associated with trauma or IMPA.

Dropped Joint

See Figures 2.28–2.32.

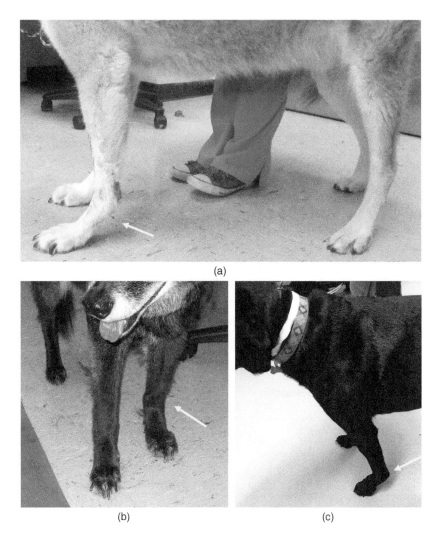

(a)

(b)　　　　　　　　　(c)

Figure 2.28　(a–c) "Dropped carpus" carpal hyperextension in a mature dog (arrows) is often associated with "jump-down" trauma causing injury to palmer fibrocartilage. This condition is different from "puppy carpal laxity syndrome" (see Figure 2.33) or erosive IMPA (see Figure 2.35). This stance is also seen in mature dogs with metacarpal-phalangeal OA.

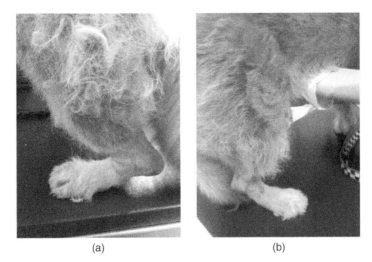

(a)   (b)

Figure 2.29 (a, b) "Dropped hock" secondary to common calcaneal (Achilles') tendon degeneration may be seen bilaterally without an acute trauma.

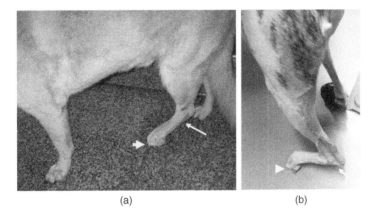

(a)   (b)

Figure 2.30 (a, b) "Dropped hock" (arrows) with "curling toe" (arrowheads) may be seen with ruptured common calcaneal (Achilles') tendon with an intact superficial digital extensor (SDF) tendon. Note that the dorsal surface of the foot is not on the ground, and this is not a "knuckling" from neurologic disorders.

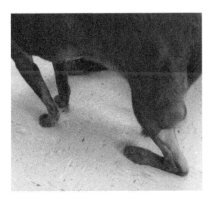

Figure 2.31 "Dropped hock" with "plantigrade stance" is commonly seen with complete rupture of common calcaneal (Achilles') tendon. This stance is also seen in dogs with intertarsal luxation.

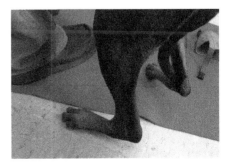

Figure 2.32 Bilateral "dropped hock" is commonly seen in specific breeds such as Doberman Pinscher with bilateral rupture of common calcaneal (Achilles') tendon.

Gross Joint Laxity

See Figures 2.33–2.35.

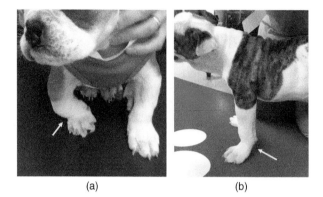

(a)   (b)

Figure 2.33 (a, b) Carpal laxity syndrome (arrows) in puppies may be associated with inadequate nutrition or poor surface in the environment.

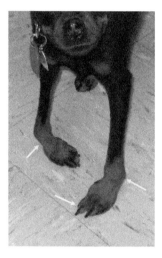

Figure 2.34 Multiple joint laxity (arrows) may be seen in puppies with congenital metabolic storage disorders such as mucopolysaccharidosis.

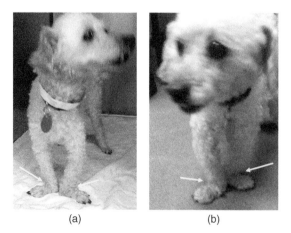

(a)   (b)

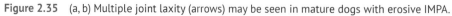

Figure 2.35 (a, b) Multiple joint laxity (arrows) may be seen in mature dogs with erosive IMPA.

2.2 Sit Observation

The dog should be examined for postural changes consistent with pelvic limb disorders, such as unwillingness to flex the knee during sitting (the "sit test") (see Figures 2.36–2.39). A "positive" sit test may suggest tarsal discomfort, but more commonly indicates stifle discomfort due to cruciate disease.

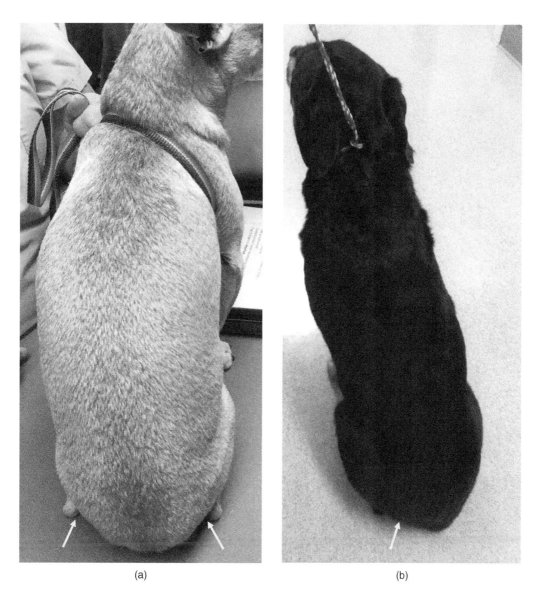

(a)   (b)

Figure 2.36 "Negative" sit test: a square sit posture with a small distance between calcaneus and tuber ischi (arrows), even with orthopedic conditions in the pelvic lims such as (a) medial patellar luxation and (b) hip dysplasia/OA.

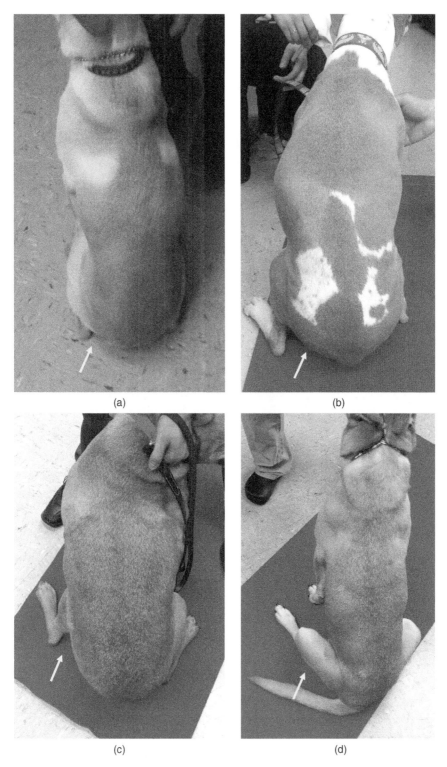

(a) (b)

(c) (d)

Figure 2.37 (a–d) "Positive" sit test: various magnitudes of noticeable distance between calcaneus and tuber ischi (arrows) can be observed. These dogs all have cruciate disease in the affected limb with a positive sit test.

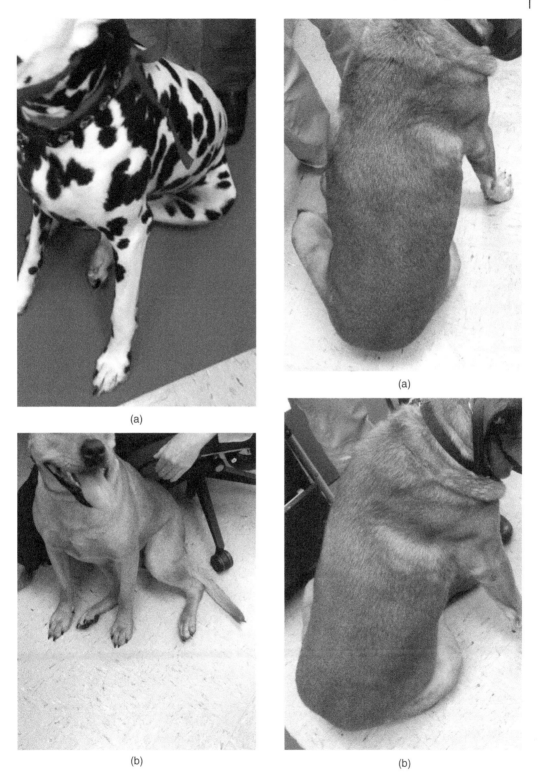

(a)

(b)

(a)

(b)

Figure 2.38 (a, b) Strong "positive" sit test: dogs do not want to sit straight due to stifle discomfort. Both dogs have cruciate disease in the affected limb with a positive sit test.

Figure 2.39 (a, b) Bilateral "positive" sit test: dogs do not want to sit straight due to stifle discomfort bilaterally. The dog has cruciate disease in both limbs.

2.3 Gait Observation

Gait visual analysis helps confirm or contradict the owner's observation (see Videos 2.1 and 2.2). Chronic lameness may disappear in an examination room, and having the owner videotape the gait at home or in a large area at the hospital is recommended. The gait is observed at a walk and a trot, from the front and back, and from the side if possible. Subtle lameness may become more apparent with tight circles or stair climbing.

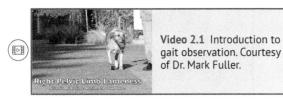

Video 2.1 Introduction to gait observation. Courtesy of Dr. Mark Fuller.

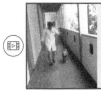

Video 2.2a Gait analysis examples. Courtesy of Dr. Koji Aoki.

Video 2.2b Gait analysis examples. Courtesy of Dr. Koji Aoki.

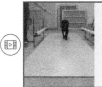

Video 2.2c Gait analysis examples. Courtesy of Dr. Koji Aoki.

Common abnormalities include:

- Systemic signs:
  - Stiff ("walking on eggshell") gait.

- Neurologic signs:
  - Stumbling, generalized weakness, ataxia, crisscrossing of the legs, hypermetria.
  - Dragging of the toenails.

- Lameness:
  - Abnormal weight bearing (non-weight bearing, toe-touching, and partial weight bearing).
  - Shortened stride.
  - Abnormal sounds (e.g., clicks, snaps).

- Head/pelvis movements:
  - Head "bob" (the head elevates as the painful thoracic limb strikes the ground).
  - Hip "hike" (the pelvic area elevates as the painful pelvic limb strikes the ground).
  - Hip "swing" (the pelvic area moves to the side as the painful pelvic limb extends).

- Abnormal gait:
  - "Toeing in" or "toeing out."
  - Limb circumduction.

Nonorthopedic causes of lameness must be ruled out first by gait observation (see Videos 2.3 and 2.4).

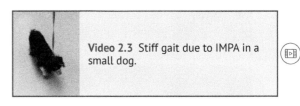

Video 2.3 Stiff gait due to IMPA in a small dog.

Video 2.4 Slow gait due to IMPA in a large dog. Courtesy of Dr. Koji Aoki.

Thoracic Limb

Orthopedic examination of thoracic limb lameness starts with observing the gait at walk.

Rule Out

Any gait abnormality suggestive of neurologic disorders must be followed by a full neurologic examination (Dewey & da Costa 2015) (see Videos 2.5–2.7). A full neurologic examination should rule out neurologic causes for pain or lameness, such as a nerve root signature sign secondary to a laterally herniated intervertebral disk or brachial plexus pathology. Non-weight-bearing or toe-touching lameness without a history of a trauma may indicate a pathologic fracture due to cancer (osteosarcoma) (see Videos 2.8–2.10).

Video 2.5 Knuckling.

Video 2.6 Brachial plexus paralysis in a small dog. Courtesy of Dr. Koji Aoki.

Video 2.7 Brachial plexus paralysis in a large dog.

Video 2.8 Severe lameness due to cancer (elbow area).

Video 2.9 Severe lameness due to cancer (shoulder area).

Video 2.10 Severe lameness due to cancer (humeral area).

Lameness

Weight-bearing lameness of the front limb typically results in a "head bob" in which the head is lifted during weight-bearing of the painful limb (see Videos 2.11–2.14). Dogs affected bilaterally may not exhibit an obvious head bob, but can show a shortened stride of each limb.

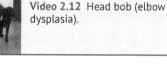

Video 2.11 Head bob (elbow dysplasia).

Video 2.12 Head bob (elbow dysplasia).

Video 2.13 Head bob (shoulder tendon disease).

Video 2.14 Head bob (biceps tendon disease).

Pelvic Limb

Orthopedic examination of the pelvic limb lameness starts with observing the gait at walk.

Rule Out

Any gait abnormality suggestive of neurologic disorders must be followed by a full neurologic examination (Dewey & da Costa 2015) (see Videos 2.15 and 2.16). A full neurologic examination should rule out neurologic causes for pain or lameness, such as a nerve root signature sign secondary to a laterally herniated intervertebral disk or lumbosacral pathology. Stiff gait may indicate a systemic condition (IMPA or Lyme disease) and lumbosacral disease (cauda-equina syndrome) (see Videos 2.17 and 2.18).

Video 2.19 Short stride gait (hip dysplasia).

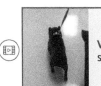
Video 2.15 Ataxic gait (congenital spinal deformity).

Video 2.20 Short stride, hip swing (hip OA).

Video 2.16 Ataxic gait (T3–L3 myelopathy).

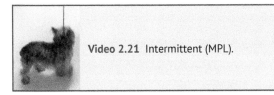
Video 2.21 Intermittent (MPL).

Video 2.17 Stiff gait (IMPA).

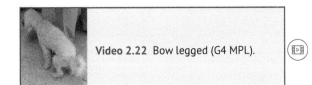
Video 2.22 Bow legged (G4 MPL).

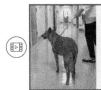
Video 2.18 Stiff gait (lumbosacral disease).

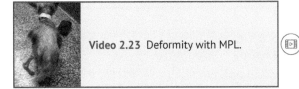
Video 2.23 Deformity with MPL.

Lameness

Pelvic limb lameness can vary in frequency from intermittent skip (such as in medial patellar luxation [MPL]) to constant lameness (such as in cranial cruciate ligament disease [CCLD]), and in severity from mild shortened stride during weight bearing (hip OA) to non-weight-bearing toe-touching (such as in cruciate disease with meniscal tear) (see Videos 2.19–2.28).

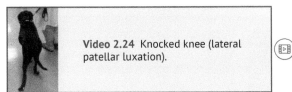
Video 2.24 Knocked knee (lateral patellar luxation).

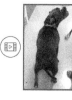

Video 2.25 Toe-touching (acute CCLD).

Video 2.27 Partial weight bearing, hip hike (CCLD).

Video 2.26 Partial weight bearing (CCLD).

Video 2.28 Toe-touching (CCLD meniscal tear).

Reference

Dewey, C.W., & da Costa, R.C. (2015). *Practical Guide to Canine and Feline Neurology*, 3rd ed. Chichester: Wiley-Blackwell.

 The videos are available for this chapter on www.wiley.com/go/hayashi/lameness.

3

Orthopedic Palpation 1: Standing Examination

Mark C. Fuller

Ideally, orthopedic patients should be palpated in both standing and recumbent positions; however, experienced veterinarians may be able to perform a thorough orthopedic examination with the patient standing. The standing examination is critical for palpation for swellings, masses, atrophy, and other abnormalities, particularly when these changes are asymmetric, such as:

- Muscle atrophy
- Elbow effusion
- Carpal effusion
- Stifle effusion
- Medial buttressing of the stifle joint
- Musculoskeletal masses
- Achilles' tendon abnormalities

Palpate deeply for pain on muscles and bone and compare from side to side while the patient is standing. The list of palpated structures is long, but a thorough standing examination can be quickly performed with experience because of the advantage of symmetric bilateral palpation. The recumbent examination may permit more thorough and easier palpation of joint range of motion, crepitus, and instability. In some situations, however, only a standing examination can be performed. Many patients will not tolerate recumbent examination because of stress, aggression, or, most commonly, hyperactivity in puppies. If the patient requires excessive restraint, perform the entire examination with the patient standing.

3.1 General and Neurologic Examination

General physical and neurologic examination must be performed with (or before) the orthopedic palpation (Figures 3.1–3.4).

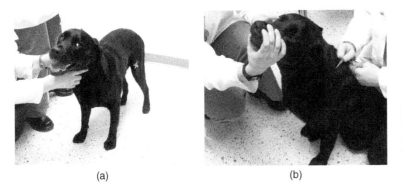

(a)   (b)

Figure 3.1 (a, b) Responsiveness and cranial nerve functions are examined (Dewey & da Costa 2015).

Diagnosis of Lameness in Dogs, First Edition. Edited by Kei Hayashi.
© 2023 John Wiley & Sons, Inc. Published 2023 by John Wiley & Sons, Inc.
Companion website: www.wiley.com/go/hayashi/lameness

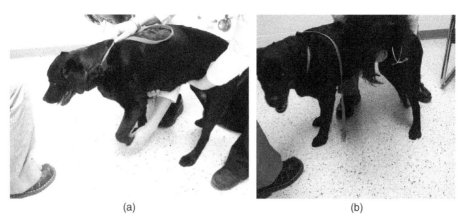

(a)   (b)

Figure 3.2   (a, b) Conscious proprioception of the leg. With the animal standing with the legs parallel, the paw is knuckled over on its dorsal aspect, while the chest or abdomen is supported. This is repeated several times. The paw should quickly right itself. A normal dog will usually not even allow the dorsum of the forepaw to be placed on the floor, unlike the rear limb (Dewey & da Costa 2015).

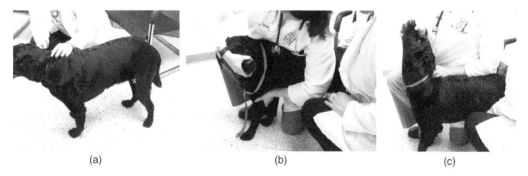

(a)   (b)   (c)

Figure 3.3   Neck palpation. (a) The neck area is gently palpated first to make sure there is no severe pain from a serious condition (such as atlantoaxial [AA] luxation or disk disease). Then the neck is flexed (b) and extended (c) to detect resistance or a painful response (Dewey & da Costa 2015).

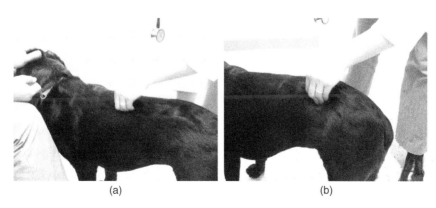

(a)   (b)

Figure 3.4   (a, b) The dorsal spines of the thoracolumbar regions are pressed downward to elicit pain (Dewey & da Costa 2015).

3.2 Thoracic Limb

Dogs bear more weight on the thoracic limbs than the pelvic limbs. Causes of lameness (and the affected anatomic locations) will differ by the age, breed (size), and lifestyle of the dog. Therefore, the orthopedic examination can focus more on areas prone to disease based on patient signalment. All anatomical aspects of the limb, however, should be assessed in every patient. For examination purposes, the thoracic limb can be anatomically divided into the shoulder/scapula, humerus (brachium), elbow, radius/ulna (antebrachium), carpal, and distal/paw regions.

As already discussed, neurologic examination should accompany orthopedic examination to rule out other sources of limb dysfunction, such as peripheral neuropathies or, more commonly, cervical intervertebral disc disease and brachial plexus disorders.

The standing examination of the thoracic limbs is often performed with the examiner standing over the patient. With the animal standing as symmetrically as possible, both hands examine the lateral aspects of the limbs simultaneously, observing for asymmetry produced by:

- Congenital defects (such as shoulder luxation, elbow luxation).

- Developmental disease (such as elbow dysplasia, shoulder osteochondrosis dissecans [OCD]).
- Trauma (such as physeal/avulsion fractures, radius/ulna fractures, carpal hyperextension).
- Neoplasia (such as osteosarcoma in proximal humerus and distal radius).
- Degenerative disease (such as elbow osteoarthritis [OA], shoulder tendinitis).

Signs to palpate are:

- Pain response on palpation and range of motion.
- Muscle atrophy/asymmetry.
- Swelling (effusion).
- Malaligned bony landmarks.
- Crepitus.

Specific landmarks to observe in the thoracic limbs are the following:

- Acromion.
- Spine of the scapula.
- Greater tubercle of the humerus.
- Humeral epicondyles associated with the elbow.
- Olecranon.
- Accessory carpal bone (located at the level of the radiocarpal joint).

Table 3.1 Examples of differentials in shoulder region (important rule-outs in italics).

	General	Small breed	Large breed
General		*Cervical lesion*	*Brachial plexus lesion*
Growing dogs	Supraglenoid fracture	Congenital shoulder luxation	Osteochondrosis dissecans
Mature dogs		Shoulder luxation	Shoulder/biceps tendinopathy *Osteosarcoma (proximal humerus)*

"Shoulder Region" (Shoulder/Scapula and Brachial Regions)

The shoulder and brachial regions are commonly affected with (Table 3.1; see also Figures 3.5 and 3.6):

- OCD.
- Supraglenoid tubercle physeal/avulsion fracture.
- Bicipital tendinitis (or rupture).
- Supraspinatus mineralization.
- Joint instability/luxation.
- Neoplasia.

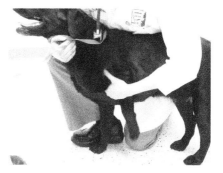

Figure 3.6 Bicipital pain may be elicited by flexing the shoulder (with elbow extension) or pressing the belly of the biceps. Supraspinatus pain may also be elicited by flexing the shoulder (less common than biceps tendinopathy).

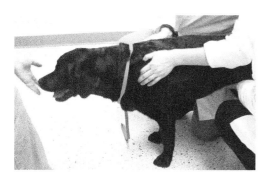

Figure 3.5 The lateral aspect is palpated. Severe muscle atrophy/asymmetry around the scapula often indicates nonorthopedic disorders (such as neoplasia or neurologic disorders). Muscle atrophy from any chronic (over 3–4 weeks) thoracic limb lameness is often detected as a more prominent acromion. The relative position and size of the acromion and greater tubercle are noted, which are altered with shoulder luxation. Severe pain on compression is noted with tumors of the proximal humerus (such as osteosarcoma).

"Elbow Region" (Elbow and Antebrachial Regions)

The elbow and antebrachial regions are commonly affected with (Table 3.2):

- Congenital luxation.
- Elbow dysplasia (medial coronoid disease – fragmentation of medial coronoid process [FCP], OCD, ununited anconeal process [UAP]).
- Incongruities/subluxation/angular limb deformities (ALD).
- Panosteitis.
- Humeral condylar fractures.
- Humeral intracondylar fissure (HIF) or incomplete ossification of the humeral condyle (IOHC).
- Luxation.
- Triceps tendon rupture.
- OA.

Table 3.2 Examples of differentials in elbow region (important rule-outs in italics).

	General	Small breed	Large breed
General	Humeral condylar fracture *Infectious (Lyme)*		
Growing dogs		Congenital luxation Incongruity/angular limb deformity (ALD)	Elbow dysplasia Incongruity/ALD *Panosteitis*
Mature dogs	*Immune-mediated poly-arthropathy (IMPA)*	Triceps tendon rupture	Elbow osteoarthritis Elbow luxation

The radius and ulnar regions are palpated for swelling and malalignment. The relationship of the carpus to the elbow should be observed as evidence of angulation (varus, valgus, procurvatum, recurvatum, or rotational or translational deformities). During the standing exam it is good to determine if there is (i) elbow joint effusion (Figure 3.7), (ii) pain on flexion or extension of the elbow, or (iii) a reduced range of motion of the elbow joint.

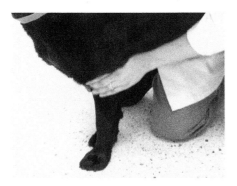

Figure 3.7 Elbow joint effusion is especially noted laterally between the lateral epicondyle of the humerus and the olecranon. Normally, only a thin anconeus muscle lies under the skin. With increased joint fluid (such as in elbow dysplasia), a bulge occurs between these two bony landmarks in the weight-bearing limb that often disappears with non-weight bearing. Osteophytes are noted (in chronic elbow dysplasia that is becoming OA) as an extra ridge lying between the epicondyle and the olecranon. Specific pain localization may be detected with medial coronoid disease by applying digital pressure over the medial coronoid.

Carpal and Paw Regions

The carpal and paw regions are commonly affected with (Table 3.3):

- Fractures/traumatic injuries (distal radius/ulna, toes).
- Hyperextension.
- Malalignment (ALD).
- Instability.
- Joint swelling (effusion due to IMPA).
- Proliferative bony changes (OA).
- Neoplasia (distal radius, nail bed).

Valgus and external rotation of the carpus are frequently seen with:

- Congenital elbow conditions (see Figure 2.2).
- Growth plate injuries (see Figure 2.18).

The dorsal carpal and metacarpal regions are palpated for swelling. The carpus and paw can be more closely evaluated by lifting the paw off the ground. Carpal range of motion can be assessed, along with swelling or discomfort associated with the metacarpal and digital regions. Further examination takes place in the recumbent examination.

Table 3.3 Examples of differentials in carpal and paw regions (important rule-outs in italics).

	General	Small breed	Large breed
General	Paw/digit injuries *Infectious (Lyme)*	Radius/ulna fractures	
Growing dogs	Puppy carpal laxity	Angular limb deformity (ALD)	ALD
Mature dogs	*Immune-mediated poly-arthropathy (IMPA)*	*Erosive IMPA*	Hyperextension *Osteosarcoma (distal radius)* *Nail bed tumor*

3.3 Pelvic Limb

Causes of lameness (and the affected anatomic locations) will differ by the age, breed (size), and lifestyle of the dog. Therefore, the orthopedic examination can focus more on areas prone to disease based on patient signalment. All anatomic aspects of the limb, however, should be assessed in every patient.

For examination purposes, the pelvic limb can be anatomically divided into the lumbosacral, hip/pelvis, femur (thigh), stifle, tibia/fibula (crus), tarsal, and distal/paw regions.

As discussed earlier, neurologic examination should accompany orthopedic examination to rule out other sources of limb dysfunction, such as peripheral neuropathies or, more commonly, intervertebral disc disease and lumbosacral disease.

With the animal standing as symmetrically as possible, both hands examine the contralateral aspects of the limbs simultaneously, observing for asymmetry produced by:

- Congenital defects.
- Developmental disease (such as hip dysplasia, femoral head necrosis, patellar luxation).
- Trauma.
- Neoplasia.
- Degenerative disease (such as hip OA, cruciate disease, common calcaneal tendinopathy).

Signs to palpate are:

- Pain response on palpation and range of motion.
- Muscle atrophy.
- Swelling (effusion).
- Malaligned bony landmarks.
- Crepitus.

Specific landmarks to observe in the pelvic limbs are:

- Iliac crests (wing) of the ilium.
- Greater trochanter.
- Ischial tuberosity.
- Extensor mechanism (quadriceps, patella, patellar tendon, and tibial tuberosity).
- Femoral condyles.
- Malleoli.

- Calcaneus.
- Common calcaneal (Achilles') tendon.

Lumbosacral Region

The lumbosacral region is commonly affected with:

- Lumbosacral disease (cauda equina syndrome).
- Anomaly (such as transitional vertebrae).
- Infection (discospondylitis).
- Lumbosacral fracture/luxation from trauma.

The dorsal aspect of the lumbosacral joint is pressed downward to elicit pain (Figure 3.8). Any abnormality suggestive of lumbosacral disease must be followed by a full neurologic examination (Dewey & da Costa 2015).

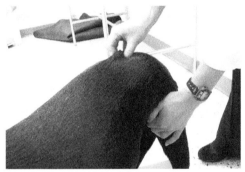
(a)

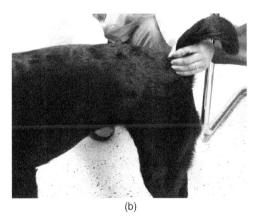
(b)

Figure 3.8 (a, b) Compression of the lumbosacral junction may elicit pain response or a sudden sitting position in dogs with lumbosacral disease. Pain response may also be elicited by lifting the tail, lordosis test, or rectal palpation (Dewey & da Costa 2015).

Table 3.4 Examples of differentials in hip region (important rule-outs in italics).

	General	Small breed	Large breed
General	Hip luxation *Infections*		
Growing dog	Physeal fracture	Femoral head necrosis	Hip dysplasia
Mature dog	*Lumbosacral disease*		Osteoarthritis Tendinopathy *Neoplasia (osteosarcoma)*

"Hip Region" (Hip/Pelvis and Thigh Regions)

The hip region and thigh regions are commonly affected with (Table 3.4):

- Hip dysplasia.
- Femoral head necrosis.
- Physeal fractures.
- Hip luxation (Figure 3.9).
- Chronic hip OA.
- Pelvic and femoral fractures from trauma.

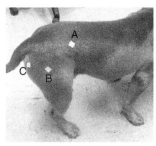

(a)

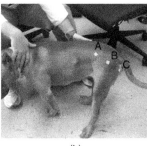

(b)

Figure 3.9 Palpate the hip region to identify three landmarks: the Iliac crests (wing) (A), greater trochanter (B), and ischial tuberosity (C). Imaginary lines are drawn connecting these three landmarks; a flat triangle should form in normal dogs. With craniodorsal hip (coxofemoral) luxation, the triangle becomes more acute (almost a straight line), with the greater trochanter more prominent at a more dorsal location.

Hip range of motion is tested for each limb individually by holding the thigh area (Figure 3.10). The muscles of the cranial and caudal thigh are palpated. Muscle atrophy from any chronic (over 3–4 weeks) pelvic limb lameness is often detected as an asymmetry at the mid-thigh area (Figure 3.11).

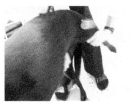

Figure 3.10 Hip extension can be tested in standing position by gently pulling the thigh caudally while holding the body with the other hand. Hip extension may elicit pain response in any disorders involving hip joint (hip luxation, hip dysplasia, femoral head necrosis, physeal fracture of the head of femur), lumbosacral joint (lumbosacral disease), and muscle disorders/tendinopathy (iliopsoas tendinopathy).

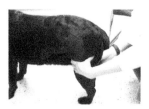

Figure 3.11 Muscle atrophy/asymmetry can be examined by placing both hands around the mid-thigh area and by comparing the left and right quickly, while the dog is bearing weight on both pelvic limbs equally. A tape measure can also be used. Muscle atrophy/asymmetry is often detected in dogs with common chronic orthopedic conditions such as cranial cruciate ligament rupture and hip dysplasia/OA. The caudal femoral region is palpated for "sciatic tract pain" (https://vetsurg.com/examinations).

Table 3.5 Examples of differentials in stifle region (important rule-outs in italics).

	General	Small breed	Large breed
General	*Infectious*	Patellar luxation	
Growing dogs	Physeal fractures		Osteochondrosis dissecans Patellar luxation
Mature dogs	Cranial cruciate ligament rupture *Immune-mediated poly-arthropathy (IMPA)*		*Osteosarcoma* *Synovial cell sarcoma*

"Stifle Region" (Stifle and Crural Regions)

The stifle and crural regions are commonly affected with (Table 3.5):

- Patellar luxation.
- OCD.
- Cranial cruciate ligament rupture.
- Femoral and tibial fractures, cruciate avulsion fractures from trauma.
- Neoplasia (osteosarcoma, synovial cell sarcoma).

Standing examination allows simultaneous palpation of the stifles bilaterally. Stifle palpation begins with locating the tibial tuberosity and following the patellar tendon proximally (Figure 3.12). Abnormal deviation of the tibial tuberosity from the midline plane should be noted as it occurs with patellar luxation.

Normal patellar tendons should be identified easily (Figure 3.13); however, joint effusion from stifle injury (such as cranial cruciate ligament rupture) makes the tendon less distinct. The patella is found 1–4 cm proximal to the tuberosity. The position of the patella is determined to identify the presence and direction of a patellar luxation (Figure 3.14). Stifle range of motion, along with assessment of the cranial tibial drawer sign and cranial tibial thrust, can be assessed during the standing and recumbent exam. The distal femur and proximal tibia are carefully palpated to rule out neoplasia in this region. The gastrocnemius muscle is palpated toward the tarsal region.

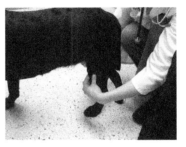

Figure 3.12 In normal dogs, the edges of the patellar tendon should be distinguished easily. Loss of palpable edges of this structure is consistent with effusion, the most common cause of which is cranial cruciate ligament rupture. Palpation of the joint just medial or lateral to the patellar tendon may elicit pain response in dogs with cranial cruciate ligament rupture. If both the stifle and tarsal joints are bilaterally effusive on standing palpation, systemic conditions (such as IMPA and Lyme disease) are suspected.

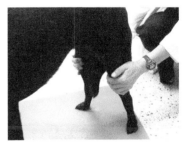

Figure 3.13 Extension of the stifle may elicit pain response in dogs with cranial cruciate ligament rupture. The proximal medial aspect of both tibias are palpated for evidence of a firm, round swelling called a fibrous "medial buttress," which occurs with chronic cranial cruciate ligament rupture. The "cranial tibial thrust test" (or "cranial drawer test") can be performed in dogs in standing position (see Chapter 4).

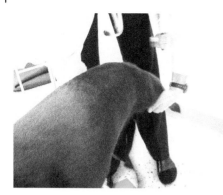

Figure 3.14 To identify dynamic patellar luxation, the examiner should stand caudal to the dog and keep the hip and stifle extended. The tibial tuberosity is located, and then the patella is identified by moving the hand proximally. Stifle and hip extension in this position may cause the patella to luxate ("pop out").

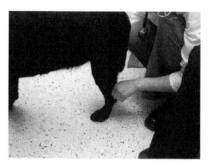

Figure 3.15 Swelling of the tarsal joint is detected on the standing dog by palpating between the malleoli and the calcaneus. Normally, only skin, subcutaneous tissue, and bone are present. Joint swelling from increased fluid accumulation (effusion) or fibrosis is detected as a firm, soft tissue mass between those two landmarks.

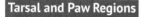
Tarsal and Paw Regions

The tarsal and paw regions are commonly affected with (Table 3.6):

- Fractures/traumatic injuries.
- OCD.
- Joint swelling (effusion due to IMPA).
- Joint swelling (OA) (Figure 3.15).
- Common calcaneal (Achilles') tendinopathy (Figure 3.16).
- Superficial digital flexor tendon dislocation.

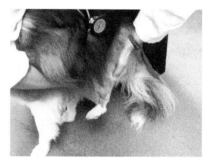

Figure 3.16 The Achilles tendon is examined above the calcaneus for swelling and continuity. Particularly in Collies and Shelties, superficial digital flexor tendon may dislocate during range of motion, which can cause lameness.

Table 3.6 Examples of differentials in tarsal and paw regions (important rule-outs in italics).

	General	Small breed	Large breed
General	Paw/digit injuries *Infectious (Lyme)*		
Growing dogs			Osteochondrosis dissecans
Mature dogs	*Immune-mediated poly-arthropathy (IMPA)*	*Erosive IMPA*	Common calcaneal tendinopathy *Osteosarcoma (distal tibia)* *Nail bed tumor*

Reference

Dewey, C.W., & da Costa, R.C. (2015). *Practical Guide to Canine and Feline Neurology*, 3rd ed. Chichester: Wiley-Blackwell.

4

Orthopedic Palpation 2: Recumbent Examination

Kimberly A. Agnello

A recumbent examination can be performed if the patient is reasonably relaxed in this position. First, assess the patient's temperament, as this may require you to alter the examination. It is important that the patient be as relaxed as possible when performing a recumbent orthopedic examination so that the examiner can have an accurate assessment of range of motion, joint stability, and pain. Stress or tension in a patient can result in nonpathologic changes in range of motion, failure to identify loss of joint stability, and false interpretation of anxiety as pain. In most situations it is best to examine the affected limb(s) last, but in some cases (particularly with active young puppies) there may only be an opportunity to palpate the diseased limb(s).

The dog is placed in lateral recumbency to further examine previously noted abnormalities by observation and standing examination. As most maneuvers do not produce pain response in normal dogs, pain response gives clues to the location of the problem. It may be best to examine the normal (non-painful) side first to learn individual responses to certain maneuvers. The signs to look for include:

- Painful regions
- Altered range of motion
- Instability
- Crepitus

In general, it is recommended to examine from the toes proximally. The known abnormal region should be examined last. Isolation of the region of interest is important (for example, when you examine the stifle, try not to move the hip or tarsal joints). Maneuvers producing pain responses should be carefully and gently repeated while immobilizing surrounding tissues to reduce the possibility of misinterpreting the origin of the pain. Laxity (of the carpal and tarsal joints) and crepitus without pain response may not be pathologic.

4.1 Thoracic Limb

Paw

Injury to the paw or digits is a frequent cause of a non-weight-bearing lameness. As many dogs are sensitive to paw palpation and tend to withdraw the limb during palpation, paw and digit palpation should be performed with other joints (carpal and elbow) in relatively flexed positions. Examination of the paw generally consists of assessing each digit, including the nail and nail bed. Common sources of lameness arising from these sites include:

- Split nails
- Nail-bed tumors
- Fracture/luxation of the phalanges
- Infection
- Penetrating foreign bodies
- Pad lacerations

Diagnosis of Lameness in Dogs, First Edition. Edited by Kei Hayashi.
© 2023 John Wiley & Sons, Inc. Published 2023 by John Wiley & Sons, Inc.
Companion website: www.wiley.com/go/hayashi/lameness

Nails are inspected for signs of wear, which may indicate digit dragging due to neurologic disorders (Figure 4.1). Careful palpation of the digits and manipulation of the joints in flexion and extension, while observing for evidence of pain or swelling, is a sensitive method to determine whether any part of the paw is a source of pain (Figure 4.2–4.5).

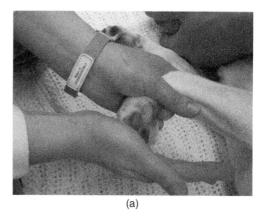

(a)

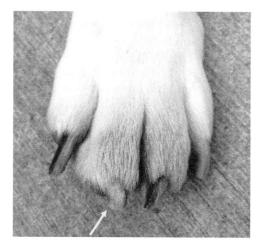

Figure 4.1 Assess the nails for wearing, which is indicative of toe dragging due to neurologic disorders. Note the wear of the nails on digits 3 (arrow) and 4 and the longer nails on digits 2 and 5.

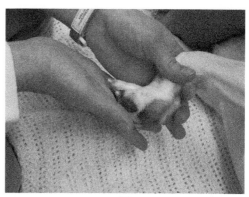

(b)

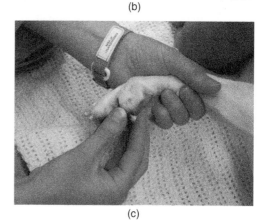

(c)

Figure 4.3 (a–c) The toe and digits are flexed, extended, and examined for trauma, swelling, and pain (suggestive signs of infection and neoplasia). Be certain to palpate each bone and the associated joints during the examination.

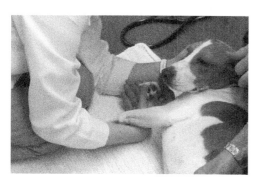

Figure 4.2 For recumbent thoracic limb examination, position yourself in front of the dog.

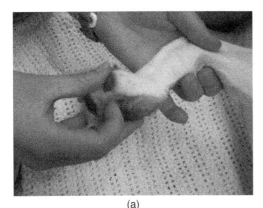

(a)

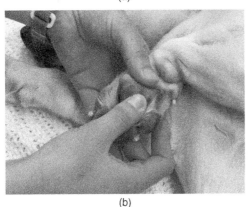

(b)

Figure 4.4 (a, b) The interdigital webbing and foot pads are examined for redness (dermatitis), laceration, abrasions, and other conditions such as a "corn."

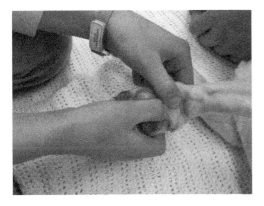

Figure 4.5 The proximal sesamoid bones are palpated for swelling on the palmar aspect of the paw at the metacarpophalangeal junction.

Carpus

Palpation of the carpus should include placing the joint under stress in extension, flexion, valgus, varus, and rotation for the observation of excessive mobility or pain in any of these planes (Figures 4.6 and 4.7). In normal dogs, the carpus should have minimal valgus and varus.

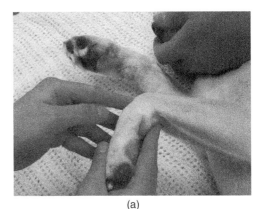

(a)

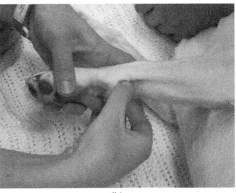

(b)

Figure 4.6 (a, b) The carpal joint space is palpated when the carpus is flexed to about 90 degrees. Swelling detected on the standing examination can be better defined when the dog is recumbent, as the exact location of the joint space can be identified. This helps to rule out joint problems (such as IMPA) from distal radial swelling seen with hypertrophic osteodystrophy (HOD) or neoplasia. The radiocarpal joint space lies at the same level as the base of the accessory carpal bone.

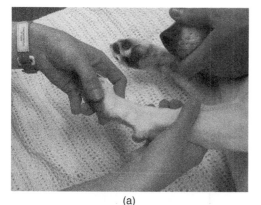

(a)

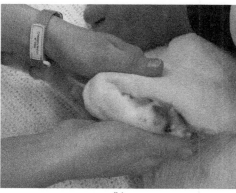

(b)

Figure 4.7 (a, b) The carpus is extended and flexed. The carpus should be able to be flexed comfortably until the palmar surface of the paw nearly touches the flexor surface of the antebrachium.

Various conditions affecting the carpus include:

- Carpal laxity syndrome in puppies
- Infection (septic arthritis)
- Immune mediate polyarthropathy (IMPA)
- Degenerative joint disease (osteoarthritis [OA])
- Subluxations or luxations from traumatic hyperextension
- Fractures

Antebrachium

Examination of the antebrachium should focus on deep palpation of both bones (radius and ulna) in an attempt to elicit an osseous source of pain or to detect focal areas of swelling (Figures 4.8 and 4.9).

Sources of lameness that can arise from the radius and ulna in young dogs include:

- HOD
- Panosteitis
- Physeal fractures/disturbances and angular limb deformities

In mature dogs they include:

- Fractures (distal radius/ulna)
- Neoplasia (distal radius)
- Hypertrophic osteopathy (HO)

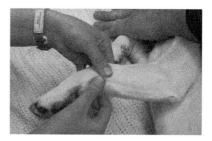

Figure 4.8 Pain detected in the distal antebrachium may indicate fracture or hypertrophic osteodystrophy in young dogs and fracture or osteosarcoma in mature dogs.

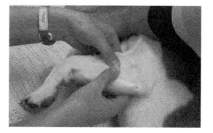

Figure 4.9 Pain detected in the proximal antebrachium may indicate panosteitis in young dogs or reflected pain from the elbow in all ages of dog.

Elbow

Recumbent examination of the elbow mainly consists of putting the joint through its range of motion in flexion and extension while observing for a painful response.

Orthopedic diseases affecting the elbow in young dogs include:

- Elbow dysplasia:
  - Medical coronoid disease, fragmented coronoid process (FCP)
  - Ununited anconeal process (UAP)
  - Osteochondosis dissecans (OCD)

- Condylar fractures
- Congenital luxations
- Incongruity (angular limb deformity [ALD])

In mature dogs they include:

- Degenerative joint disease (OA)
- Fractures/Luxations
- Neoplasia

Hyperextension or full flexion of the elbow may produce pain in dogs with elbow dysplasia. Internal and external rotation with digital pressure applied at the medial joint line may produce pain in dogs with medial coronoid disease (Figures 4.10 and 4.11). Range of motion is usually limited in dogs with elbow OA.

The rotational stability (pronation of the elbow averages 30° and supination 50°) and integrity of the collateral ligaments can be tested with the carpus and elbow at 90° (Campbell's test).

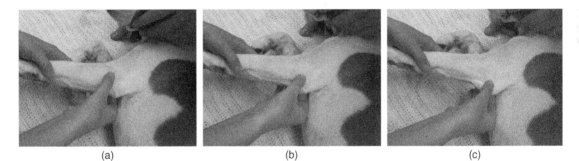

(a)	(b)	(c)

Figure 4.10 (a–c) Elbow joint effusion can be palpated by digitally feeling both (medial and lateral) distal humeral epicondyles simultaneously with index finger and thumb, while drawing fingers caudally toward the olecranon. Normally, there is a concave depression between these structures. With effusion, however, this area can become distended. With chronicity of abnormality, there may be thickening of joint capsule and osteophytosis, which can be palpated more firmly.

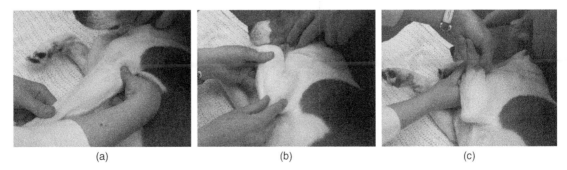

(a)	(b)	(c)

Figure 4.11 (a–c) The elbow is placed through a range of motion. Hyperextension should be accompanied by only minimal or no discomfort in a normal dog. At full elbow flexion, the space between carpal and shoulder joints should be 1–2 fingers distance.

Brachium

Examination of the brachium essentially consists of deep palpation along the length of the bone to examine for evidence of pain and areas of swelling (Figure 4.12).

Conditions potentially affecting the canine brachium in young dogs include:

- Panosteitis
- Fractures

In the adult dog they include:

- Fractures
- Neoplasia

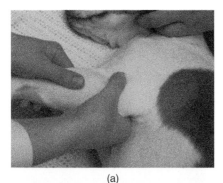

(a)

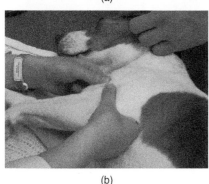

(b)

Figure 4.12 (a, b) Pain in the distal humeral region in young dogs may indicate panosteitis. Pain in the proximal humeral region in mature dogs may indicate bone tumor. Osteosarcoma commonly affects the proximal humerus and distal radius and ulna.

Shoulder

Recumbent examination of the shoulder joint is performed by putting the joint through a full range of motion to observe for excessive excursion, or elicitation of pain in any particular direction. For example, the joint should be comfortably flexed and extended, internally and externally rotated, and abducted and adducted.

Young dogs with shoulder pain should be examined closely for:

- OCD
- Congenital shoulder luxation (with glenoid dysplasia)
- Ununited caudal accessory process of the glenoid
- Fractures

In the adult dog common sources of lameness localized to the shoulder can include:

- Shoulder tendinopathy:
  - Biceps tenosynovitis
  - Supraspinatus mineralization
  - Infraspinatus contracture

- Shoulder instability or luxations
- Fractures
- Degenerative joint disease (OA)

The biceps tendon should be palpated as it originates on the supraglenoid tuberosity and courses down the intertubercular groove for evidence of inflammation. Deep digital pressure is applied to the biceps tendon, while flexing the shoulder and extending the elbow in an attempt to elicit pain as supportive evidence for biceps tenosynovitis. Shoulder instability may be appreciated in the sedated or anesthetized patient by applying a mediolateral or craniocaudal sliding motion at the joint level (Figures 4.13–4.16).

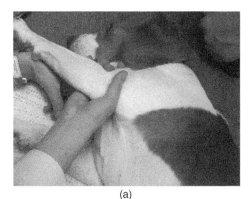

(a)

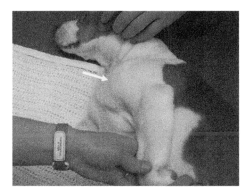

(b)

Figure 4.13 (a, b) The shoulder is examined for pain by flexing and extending the joint while grasping the brachium (not the antebrachium). OCD usually produces pain with this maneuver. Swelling or effusion of the shoulder joint unfortunately cannot be appreciated because of its depth under musculature.

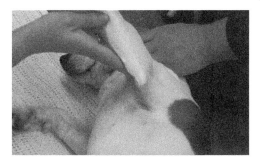

Figure 4.14 Bicipital tendinopathy or rupture is painful when the tendon is stretched or placed under tension. To produce diagnostic discomfort, the shoulder is fully flexed and the elbow is extended, where the entire limb is pulled caudally along the thoracic wall. Additionally, digital pressure can be applied to the proximal medial humeral region over the tendon (arrow) to elicit pain.

Figure 4.15 A shoulder abduction can be performed to test the medial instability and integrity of the medial joint capsule, collateral ligament, and subscapularis tendon. The angle between the scapula and humerus is measured during abduction. Comparing the abduction angle to the other limb may help establish its significance.

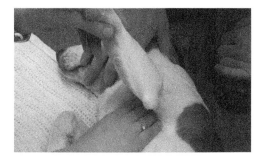

Figure 4.16 The medial aspect of the shoulder joint is palpated to detect pain from brachial plexus pathology such as a peripheral nerve sheath tumor.

Scapula

Examination of the scapula should focus on palpation of bone in an attempt to elicit an osseous source of pain or to detect focal areas of swelling due to fracture (such as avulsion fracture of supraglenoid tubercle) or neoplasia (Figure 4.17). Furthermore, the supraspinatus and infraspinatus muscles and prominence of the interposed acromial spine should be felt for muscle atrophy, as that is evidence of many neurologic/neoplastic conditions. The muscular attachment of the scapula can also be avulsed from the thoracic wall with certain types of trauma. Scapular dislocation is primarily diagnosed by palpation of excessive excursion of the scapula from the chest wall, since radiographs can look deceptively normal.

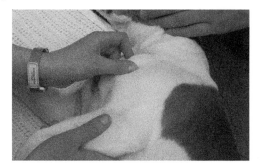

Figure 4.17 The acromion and spine of the scapula can be easily palpated. Fractures and neoplasia will cause pain on palpation.

4.2 Pelvic Limb

Paw

Injury to the paw or digits is a frequent cause of a non-weight-bearing lameness. As many dogs are sensitive to paw palpation and tend to withdraw the limb during palpation, paw and digit palpation should be performed with other joints (tarsal and stifle) in relatively flexed positions. Examination of the paw generally consists of assessing each digit, including the nail and nail bed.

Common sources of lameness arising from these sites include:

- Split nails
- Nail-bed tumors
- Fracture/luxation of the phalanges
- Infection
- Penetrating foreign bodies
- Pad lacerations

Nails are inspected for signs of wearing, which may indicate toe dragging due to neurologic disorders. Careful palpation of the digits and manipulation of the joints in flexion and extension, while observing for evidence of pain or swelling, is a sensitive method to determine whether any part of the paw is a source of pain (see Figures 4.1–4.3, 4.18 and 4.19).

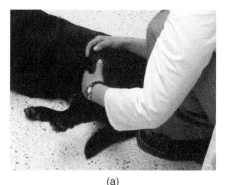

(a)

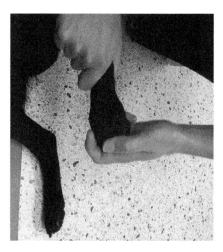

(b)

Figure 4.18 (a, b) For recumbent pelvic limb examination, position yourself behind the dog.

Figure 4.19 The digits and paw are examined similar to the thoracic limb. Assess the nails for wearing, which is indicative of toe dragging due to neurologic disorders. The toe and digits are flexed, extended, and examined for trauma, swelling, and pain (suggestive signs of infection and neoplasia). The interdigital webbing and foot pads are examined for redness (dermatitis), laceration, abrasions, and other conditions such as a "corn."

Tarsus (Hock)

The tarsal joint should be palpated for swelling/effusion, range of motion in flexion and extension, and stressed in medial and lateral directions (varus and valgus angles) to assess for excessive laxity (Figures 4.20–4.22).

Conditions potentially affecting the canine tarsus in young dogs include:

- OCD of the talus
- Fractures

In the adult dog they include:

- Common calcaneal (Achilles') tendinopathy
- Tendon and ligament breakdown (seen especially in Collies and Shelties)
- Fractures
- Polyarthropathy (such as IMPA)

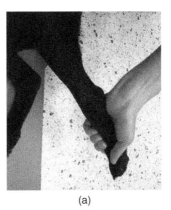

(a)

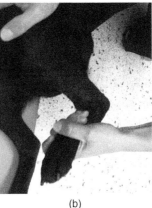

(b)

Figure 4.21 (a, b) The tarsal joint should be palpated for swelling/effusion, and for range of motion in flexion and extension. Through its normal range of motion, "popping" can occur with displacement of the superficial digital flexor tendon, especially in Collies and Shelties.

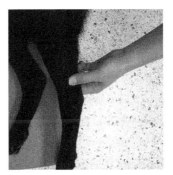

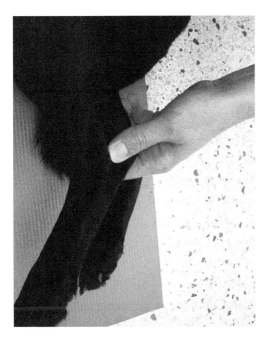

Figure 4.20 Swelling of the tarsal joint can be detected by palpating between the malleoli and the calcaneus. Normally, only skin, subcutaneous tissue, and bone are present. Young large-breed dogs should be examined closely for swelling in the tibiotarsal joint, which may be consistent with OCD. Distension of the joint capsule is palpable on the dorsal surface, as well as caudomedial and caudolateral aspects. Joint swelling in adult dogs may be attributable to degenerative joint disease or the various causes of suppurative arthritis (such as IMPA or Lyme disease).

Figure 4.22 Achilles' tendon continuity is palpated during flexion and extension of the tarsocrural joint. Common cause of a "dropped hock" or hyperflexed tibiotarsal joint is damage to the common calcaneal (Achilles') tendon. This structure should be palpated from its insertion on the calcaneus proximally to assess for disruption, swelling, pain, or fibrosis associated with injury. Displacement of the superficial digital flexor tendon occurs with associated retinaculum tearing.

Tibia and Fibula

Sources of lameness in young dogs that can arise from the tibia and fibula include:

- Panosteitis
- HOD
- Salter–Harris fractures and physeal disturbances

In both young adult and adult dogs they include:

- Fractures
- Neoplasia
- ALD
- HO

Examination of the tibia should focus on deep palpation to elicit an osseus source of pain or detect focal areas of swelling (Figure 4.23).

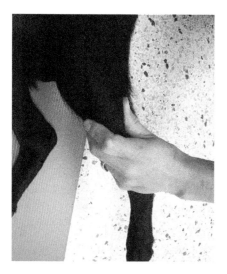

Figure 4.23 Pain in the tibia in young dogs may indicate physeal fractures or panosteitis. Pain in the proximal and distal regions in mature dogs may indicate bone tumor. Osteosarcoma commonly affects the proximal tibia, distal femur, and distal tibia.

Note that the saphenous nerve runs obliquely (along with the cranial branch of the medial saphenous artery and vein), across the proximal to mid-tibial diaphysis, therefore do not misinterpret a pain response when palpating this area as osseus bone pain. The relationship of the tarsus to the stifle should also be observed for evidence of angulation from physeal damage and abnormal development of the tibia and fibula. Aberrant growth from physeal disturbances can result in varus, valgus, procurvatum, recurvatum, or rotational or translational deformities.

Stifle

Recumbent examination of the stifle can typically begin with putting the joint through its full range of motion, which should be easily accomplished without pain in normal dogs. Pain at full extension or limited flexion may indicate cruciate disease. Patellar luxation may occur during normal range of motion. Clicking or popping may indicate chronic OA or meniscal tears secondary to cruciate disease.

In young dogs the stifle joint is often affected with:

- Luxating patellas
- OCD
- Avulsion of ligaments and tendons
- Physeal fractures of the distal femur or proximal tibia

In mature dogs conditions include:

- Cruciate disease (including meniscal tear and OA)
- Poly-arthropathy such (as IMPA and Lyme disease)
- Neoplasia

The most common cause of joint swelling (effusion) is cruciate disease. With fracture, the stifle is quite swollen, with a history of young animals sustaining trauma. Swelling (effusion) also occurs with OCD in young dogs and inflammatory joint conditions (such as IMPA) in mature dogs. Localized swelling occurs with avulsion of the origin of the long digital extensor tendon.

The patella should be assessed with the dog in lateral recumbency through normal range of motion, and while the tibia is rotated both internally and externally, to determine whether medial or lateral laxity is present (Figures 4.24 and 4.25).

The integrity of the cranial cruciate ligament is examined through an "active" cranial tibial thrust maneuver and a "passive" cranial drawer test (Figures 4.26 and 4.27). The stifle should then be placed under stress both medially and laterally (valgus and varus) to assess both collateral ligaments (Figure 4.28). Increased drawer movement occurs with multiple ligament tears in the traumatized animal or in cushingoid dogs. If there is patellar luxation, the patella should be reduced if possible before examining for cruciate instability.

Meniscal injury is suspected when the animal has a non-weight-bearing lameness several weeks after acute onset of stifle lameness, or when the owner hears a click when the animal walks. In addition, worsening of an improving lameness several weeks to months after cruciate rupture with or without surgical repair sometimes indicates meniscal involvement.

Patellar Luxation
Luxation of the patella out of the trochlea of the femur (groove) is abnormal and can cause lameness. Luxation may be medial, or less often lateral, and occasionally in both directions. Luxation of a patella is normally not a painful maneuver. There is some normal mediolateral movement within the trochlea in some dogs (Figures 4.24 and 4.25). Subluxation (patella rides on the trochlear ridge, and "catches" during flexion) occasionally causes lameness.

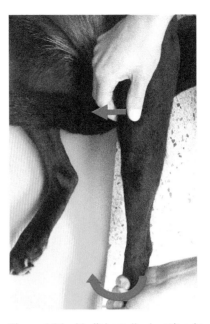

Figure 4.24 Medial patellar luxation. An unstable patella may be luxated simply by internally rotating the paw (curved arrow). To luxate a reduced patella medially, the stifle (and hip and tarsus) is extended, the toes are internally rotated, and digital pressure (thumb) is applied to the patella in a medial direction (arrow).

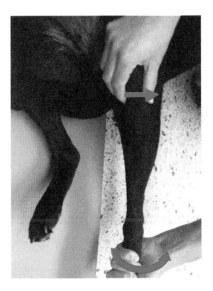

Figure 4.25 Lateral patellar luxation. An unstable patella may be luxated simply by externally rotating the paw (curved arrow). To luxate a reduced patella laterally, the stifle is flexed slightly, toes are externally rotated, and digital pressure (index finger) is applied in a lateral direction (arrow).

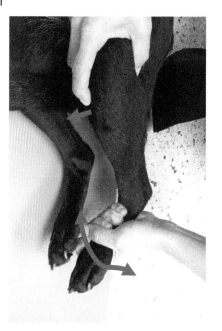

Figure 4.26 "Cranial thrust" (tibial compression) test. The stifle is held at a fixed "standing" angle and the hock is dorsi-flexed quicky and then relaxed (curved arrow), while the index finger of the opposite hand lies cranial to the femur, patellar ligament, and tibial tuberosity, palpating for cranial subluxation of the proximal tibia at the level of the tibial tuberosity (arrow). It is repeated several times quickly but gently. Interpretation of this maneuver is more subjective than direct drawer movement, but it has the advantage of producing minimal pain in animals with ruptured cranial cruciate ligaments.

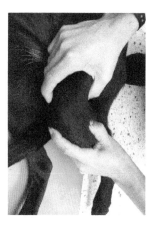

Figure 4.27 "Drawer" test. Direct drawer movement is evaluated by placing the fingers on specific boney landmarks to avoid any confusion of movement from the soft tissues. The index finger of one hand is placed on the cranial proximal patellar region, while the thumb is placed caudally on the lateral fabella. The index finger of the opposite hand is placed on the cranial aspect of the tibial crest, while the thumb is positioned caudally on the fibular head. With the wrists held straight and not bent, the femur is held stable while the tibia is pushed forward (and not rotated), then pulled backward. This is repeated quickly and gently several times. First, the stifle is held firmly in slight extension (standing angle), and then the movement repeated with the stifle held in flexion. In large dogs it is helpful to have an assistant or the examiner's foot (if performed on the floor) to support the dog's limb when performing this test.

Noting the location of the tibial tuberosity helps to differentiate a medial luxation that is reduced into the trochlea and a reduced patella that can be luxated laterally. In small dogs with ectopic patella, the patella is palpated as a small, "pealike" bump on the medial (or lateral) femoral condyle, and it may or may not move with flexion, extension, and digital pressure.

Cruciate Disease

Palpation for cruciate ligament instability can produce pain and should be performed gently in the relaxed patient. Sedation may be needed if no abnormality can be detected in the tense animal. The stifle should be examined for cruciate ligament instability with the patella reduced if possible.

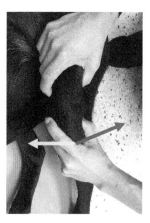

Figure 4.28 Collateral ligament instability. When the collateral ligaments *and* joint capsule are torn, the stifle will have medial (valgus), lateral (varus), or combined instability. The cruciate ligament(s) is (are) invariably torn in many clinical cases of collateral instability. To detect this instability, the stifle should be held in "neutral" drawer while a valgus (medial opening) (red arrow) or varus (lateral opening) (yellow arrow) force is applied.

The integrity of the cranial cruciate ligament can be examined through a cranial tibial thrust maneuver and a passive cranial drawer test (Figures 4.26 and 4.27); however, these tests are subjective and insensitive to cruciate disease. Factors contributing to the inaccuracy of these tests include:

- Technical error (not performing the test correctly)
- Stable stifle with small partial ligament tear
- Chronicity of cruciate disease (periarticular fibrosis, osteophytosis)
- Animal tenseness (resistance)
- Age ("puppy drawer" is normal)
- Size (large dogs show relatively small instability compared with small dogs)
- Presence of a meniscal injury ("wedged-in" effect)

Drawer movement is the cranial sliding or translation of the tibia in relation to the femur. In normal mature dogs, there is no cranial or caudal drawer movement, therefore a positive drawer test means the cranial cruciate ligament is not intact or is nonfunctional. Some rotary motion of the tibia is normal and is occasionally mistaken as drawer movement. Large puppies have normal "puppy" drawer, which lasts up to 10–12 months of age. "Puppy" drawer has a sudden end point cranially and caudally. With cranial cruciate ligament rupture, the cranial end point of the drawer test is "soft," with no sudden stoppage. When the tibia is pulled caudally, a sudden "thud" is palpated as the normal caudal cruciate ligament becomes taut. Conversely, with rare caudal cruciate ligament rupture, when cranial force is applied there is a sudden "thud" that is not present when caudal force is applied.

Meniscal injury is suspected when a "meniscal click" is produced during stifle range of motion and/or when performing the thrust and drawer tests. A definitive diagnosis of a meniscal injury is made by direct visualization, via arthroscopy or arthrotomy, of the torn portion of the meniscus or when the unstable torn segment is malpositioned within the joint.

Femur

Examination of the femur should include deep palpation along the length of the femur to examine for pain or swelling (Figures 4.29 and 4.30).

Conditions potentially affecting the femur in the young dog include:

- Panosteitis
- Fractures

In the adult dog they include:

- Fractures
- Neoplasia

A common tumor of the canine rear limb is osteosarcoma, which more frequently forms in the distal femur and proximal tibia.

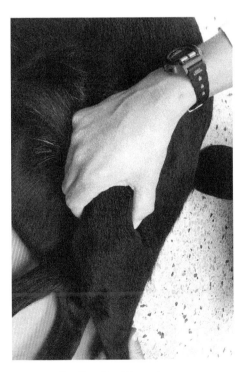

Figure 4.29 The distal femur is a common location for panosteitis and physeal fractures in young dogs, and osteosarcoma in mature dogs. It is also a region of the femur bone that is readily palpated due to less soft tissue coverage.

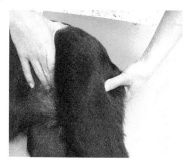

Figure 4.30 The caudal femoral region is palpated for "sciatic tract pain" (https://vetsurg.com/examinations).

Hip

A recumbent examination of the hip starts by placing the joint through the full range of motion, including flexion and extension, abduction and adduction, while observing for pain or palpable crepitus (Figures 4.31–4.33).

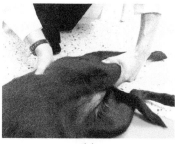

(a)

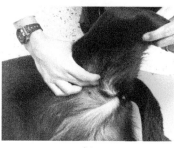

(b)

Figure 4.31 (a, b) Manipulations may cause pain, crepitus, and instability in dogs with hip disorders. The femur is grasped at or above the stifle, and the hip is flexed, extended, and abducted several times. If pain or crepitus is not produced, external hip rotation is added to the flexion and extension maneuvers. This maneuver frequently elicits pain in the animal with femoral head necrosis. Abduction and palpation of the pectineus region may elicit pain in chronic hip OA.

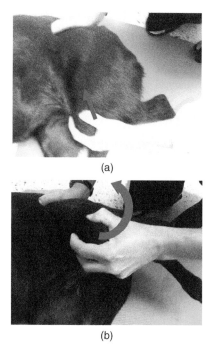

(a)

(b)

Figure 4.32 (a, b) Hip laxity seen with hip dysplasia in young dogs may be detected by the Ortolani test, which evaluates the quality and quantity of hip "reduction" during abduction, after forced hip "subluxation." To perform this, it is easiest in lateral recumbency and the dog will likely require light sedation. The stifle and hip should both be at 90° of flexion. A compressive force is applied along the axis of the femur (arrow), with one hand at the level of the stifle, while a counter-compressive force is applied over the hip and pelvis with the opposite hand. If hip laxity is present, the femoral head will have subluxated slightly during this phase. While the axial force is applied, the leg is abducted slowly (curved arrow) and the Ortolani sign is sought: a palpable clunk signifying the reduction of the head into the acetabulum. This can also be done bilaterally with the dog in dorsal recumbency. The stifles are adducted, pushed proximally, and then abducted to produce the positive Ortolani sign. This maneuver is often painful even in normal animals.

The dog with hip luxation will not allow these maneuvers due to pain (Figure 4.34).

Causes of pain in the canine hip of the young animal include:

- Hip dysplasia with laxity (subluxation)
- Avascular necrosis of femoral head (Legg–Calvé–Perthes disease)
- Luxations
- Physeal fractures

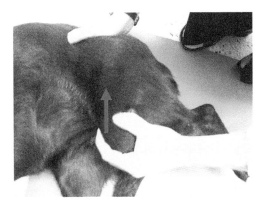

Figure 4.33 Hip laxity seen with hip dysplasia in young dogs may be detected by Barden's test. Place the dog in lateral recumbency. One palm stabilizes the pelvis, while the other hand grasps the distal femur and positions it parallel to the table or floor. The femoral head is alternately levered laterally and relaxed (arrow). The amount of subluxation may be detected. This maneuver is often painful even in normal animals.

In the adult dog they include:

- Degenerative joint disease (OA) secondary to hip dysplasia
- Luxations
- Femoral neck fracture
- Iliopsoas tendinopathy (Figure 4.35).
- Refereed pain from lumbosacral disease

Young dogs may be examined for hip laxity as a sign of the early phase of canine hip dysplasia. Although many palpation maneuvers exist, one of the most common techniques is the Ortolani examination (Figures 4.32 and 4.33).

Suspected fracture and dislocation are further evaluated by radiography. The sacroiliac joint is examined for instability by gentle manipulation of the wing of the ilium. The ischial tuberosity is pressed to detect instability and crepitus. A rectal examination may detect pubic and ischial fractures.

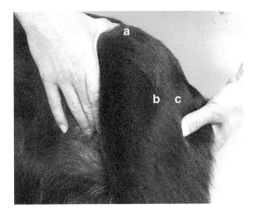

Figure 4.34 Hip luxation may be detected by identifying three landmarks: the Iliac crests (wing) of the ilium (a), greater trochanter (b), and ischial tuberosity (c). Imaginary lines are drawn connecting these three landmarks; a flat triangle should form in normal dogs. With craniodorsal hip luxation, the triangle becomes more acute (almost a straight line), with the greater trochanter more prominent at a more dorsal location (arrow). The "thumb compression" test can also be performed to detect dorsal hip luxation. Place a thumb between the greater trochanter and ischial tuberosity while the femur is externally rotated by the other hand. If the hip is luxated, the thumb will feel no pressure and remain in its location between the greater trochanter and the ischium.

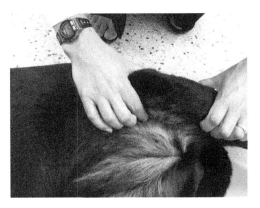

Figure 4.35 Iliopsoas tendinopathy may be detected by placing the iliopsoas musculotendinous complex under tension and assessing for a pain response. This is accomplished by extending the hip and internally rotating the femur. In addition, while placing the iliopsoas under tension one can directly compress its tendinous insertion on the femur at the lesser trochanter; however, the results can be misinterpreted, as direct compression on the femoral nerve in this location may elicit a pain response in normal dogs.

Pelvis/Lumbosacral Region

Painful conditions of the pelvis include:

- Lumbosacral disease (Figure 4.36).
- Fractures
- Luxations of the sacroiliac joint
- Neoplasia

Palpation of the pelvis can be paired with palpation of the proximal femur. The appropriate relationship between pelvis and femur can be documented by the palpation of the wing of the ilium, ischial tuberosity, and greater trochanter, which should form a triangle (Figure 4.34). Most pelvic fractures will be definitively diagnosed by using radiographs and/or computed tomography scan, but they may first be detected through palpation. The rectal palpation will allow assessment of lumbosacral pain, as well as the ventral pubic symphysis and medial walls of the acetabulum, depending on the size of the dog.

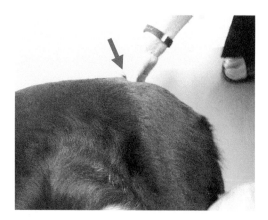

Figure 4.36 The lumbosacral region should be palpated with the hip flexed to distinguish pain due to hip extension (arrow). Direct compression of the lumbosacral junction may elicit pain response in dogs with lumbosacral disease. Pain response may also be elicited by lifting the tail, lordosis test, or rectal palpation (Dewey & da Costa 2015).

Reference

Dewey, C.W., & da Costa, R.C. (2015). *Practical Guide to Canine and Feline Neurology*, 3rd ed. Chichester: Wiley-Blackwell.

Section 2

Common Orthopedic Conditions

5

Thoracic Limb Conditions

Kimberly A. Agnello

5.1 Common General Conditions

Panosteitis

Young Large Breed

Panosteitis predominantly affects rapidly growing large-breed dogs.

- Young dogs (<2 years of age) are most commonly affected; however, it has occasionally been diagnosed in older dogs.
- German Shepherds have a higher risk of developing this disease than other large-breed dogs.

History
- Shifting leg lameness associated with pain on deep bone palpation.
- Although initial episodes of panosteitis may present as acute lameness in a single limb, the typical history consists of chronic, intermittent, shifting leg lameness.

Physical Examination
- Affected dogs are commonly lame in only a single limb.
- Firm palpation of affected long bones usually elicits pain.

Diagnostic Imaging
- The radiographic signs include blurring of trabecular patterns, followed by the appearance of radiopaque, patchy, or mottled bone within medullary canals (Figure 5.1).
- Radiographs of affected limbs can be normal during early stages, and clinical signs may precede radiographic abnormalities by up to 10 days. If clinical signs are consistent with panosteitis, but radiographs are normal, radiographs should be repeated in 7–10 days.

Idiopathic Immune-Mediated Polyarthritis

Adult Small/Large Breed

Idiopathic nonerosive inflammatory arthropathies such as idiopathic immune-mediated polyarthritis (IMPA) have no identifiable cause and are diagnosed by ruling out all other causes of polyarthritis, septic arthritis, rickettsial arthritis, rheumatoid arthritis, other inflammatory nonerosive polyarthropathies, and osteoarthritis.

- IMPA is diagnosed by synovial fluid analysis and negative culture, by joint radiographs that do not show erosive or proliferative bone lesions, and by eliminating other known causes.

Diagnosis of Lameness in Dogs, First Edition. Edited by Kei Hayashi.
© 2023 John Wiley & Sons, Inc. Published 2023 by John Wiley & Sons, Inc.
Companion website: www.wiley.com/go/hayashi/lameness

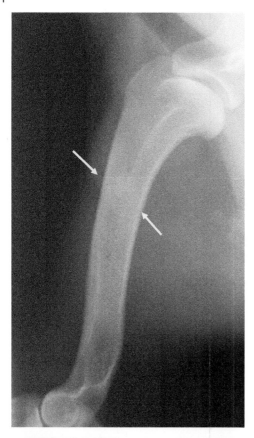

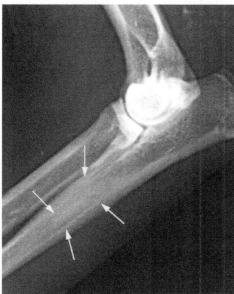

Figure 5.1 Examples of radiographs indicating panosteitis (arrows).

- A therapeutic trial of antibiotics is sometimes used to help eliminate occult infectious causes.
- All breeds and ages of dogs are susceptible to IMPA.
- Some studies have suggested breed predilections in German Shepherds, Doberman Pinschers, Collies, Spaniels, Retrievers, Terriers, and Poodles. Females are more commonly affected.

History
- Stiffness, difficulty rising, pyrexia, anorexia, and/or lethargy may be present.
- Although more than one joint is usually involved, single-limb lameness is common.
- Affected animals may or may not have difficulty rising and walking.
- Some animals have a chronic fever of unknown origin.

Physical Examination
- Joint palpation may reveal pain, effusion, or loss of range of motion.
- However, palpable joint effusion may be absent.

Diagnostic Imaging
- Radiographs of affected joints usually reveal either no abnormalities or synovial fluid effusion and periarticular soft tissue swelling (see Section 5.7).

Laboratory Findings
- Nucleated cell counts in joint fluid are notably elevated, with predominantly non-degenerative neutrophils.

Erosive IMPA (Rheumatoid Arthritis)

Adult Small/Large Breed

Rheumatoid arthritis is an erosive, noninfectious, inflammatory joint disease characterized by chronic, bilaterally symmetric, erosive destruction of the joints.

- The etiology of rheumatoid arthritis is unknown, but it is considered an immune-mediated arthropathy.
- Diagnosis of classic rheumatoid arthritis requires the presence of destructive lesions seen radiographically.
- Rheumatoid arthritis can affect any breed of dog, but it is primarily found in adults, usually greater than 5 years old.

History
- Most affected dogs have a history of stiffness after rest, limping, or difficulty walking.
- Unstable joints may be obvious.

Physical Examination
- In chronic cases, joints are generally enlarged, with periarticular soft tissue swelling and joint effusion.
- The distal joints (i.e., carpi and tarsi) may be unstable, with obvious deformity and angulation.

Diagnostic Imaging
- Radiographs of the joints show a generalized loss of mineralization, radiolucent foci, and irregular joint margins (see Section 5.7).
- Bone proliferation may also be present. Soft tissue swelling and joint effusion may be evident.

Laboratory Findings
- Joint fluid nucleated cell counts are greatly elevated, with predominantly nondegenerative neutrophils.

Septic Arthritis
Any Age, Any Breed

Septic arthritis (infective arthritis, suppurative arthritis) is joint infection caused by bacterial organisms.

- Septic arthritis may be due to hematogenous spread of infection from respiratory, digestive, urinary, umbilical, or valvular infections, but more often it is caused by direct bacterial inoculation of joints from penetrating trauma (e.g., cat bite), surgical procedures, or intra-articular injections.
- Diagnosis of septic arthritis is based on synovial fluid analysis and positive results on bacterial culture.
- Osteoarthritis (OA) is known to increase the risk of septic arthritis in people and likely increases the risk in dogs.
- Diseases such as chronic hip OA may increase the risk of septic arthritis, and this diagnosis should be considered when examining patients with severe hip pain and OA.

Signalment
- Septic arthritis can be found in any aged dog, but males of larger breeds are more commonly affected.

History
- Penetrating wounds, surgical intervention, or joint injection are often historical findings.

Physical Examination
- Animals with acute onset of signs are often severely lame or non-weight bearing on the affected limb.
- The affected joint may be swollen, painful, warm, and crepitate; drain purulent material; and have reduced range of motion.
- Systemic signs (pyrexia, lethargy, and anorexia) occur in a small percentage of animals with septic arthritis.
- The signs may be subtle (i.e., only lameness and joint swelling) with low-grade, chronic infections.

Diagnostic Imaging
- Early radiographic signs of septic arthritis are joint effusion and soft tissue swelling.
- Later changes include bone lysis, periosteal new bone formation, joint surface irregularities, subchondral bone sclerosis, and joint subluxation.

Osteomyelitis

Any Age, Any Breed

Osteomyelitis is an inflammation of bone due to infection.

- Most bone infections in dogs are bacterial in origin.
- Bacterial osteomyelitis is often classified as hematogenous or post-traumatic; however, the former is rarely reported in dogs.
- Mycotic bone infections are acquired through hematogenous dissemination of inhaled spores.
- Although viral osteomyelitis is considered uncommon, newer evidence suggests that it may occur more frequently.
- Diagnosis of osteomyelitis is often suspected on the basis of history, clinical signs, and radiographic findings.
- Any age, breed, or sex of dog or cat may be affected.

History
- Historical findings may include bite wounds, open traumatic wounds, or habitation in an endemic fungal region; however, fungal osteomyelitis must never be eliminated simply because the patient does not live in an endemic area.

Physical Examination
- Clinical features of osteomyelitis vary depending on the stage of the disease.
- The initial response of bone to infection is inflammation; soft tissue in the area can become hot, reddened, swollen, and painful.
- The animal is often pyrexic, depressed, and partially or totally anorexic.

Diagnostic Imaging
- Specific radiographic findings vary depending on the stage of disease, site of infection, and pathogenicity of infective organisms.
- Soft tissue swelling is the first sign of acute osteomyelitis and may be observed.
- Early radiographic changes include periosteal proliferation with deposition of new bone in a lamellar pattern oriented perpendicular to the long axis of the bone.

Laboratory Findings
- With acute osteomyelitis, systemic evidence of infection is often present, which is typically indicated by an elevated white blood cell count and neutrophilia with or without a left shift. Laboratory analysis in dogs with chronic osteomyelitis is usually normal. Microbiologic culturing is definitive for bacterial osteomyelitis and is essential in determining the organism's in vitro susceptibility to antimicrobial drugs.
- Fungal cultures and cytologic or histologic evaluation of biopsies may be diagnostic of fungal osteomyelitis.

Other Poly-Arthropathies

Any Age, Any Breed

Rickettsial/Anaplasmal Polyarthritis

Polyarthritis may be caused by obligate intracellular microorganisms of the families Rickettsiales (i.e., *Rickettsia rickettsii*) and Anaplasmataceae (i.e., *Ehrlichia* spp., *N. risticii*, *A. phagocytophilum*).

- Any breed of dog of any age can be affected. Dogs that are exposed to ticks (e.g., hunting dogs) may be more likely to become infected.

Lyme Arthropathy

Lyme arthropathy is a form of polyarthritis caused by *B. burgdorferi*.

- Dogs of any age or breed may be affected. Dogs that are in endemic areas and are exposed to ticks are most likely to be infected.
- Dogs with Lyme disease can have acute fever, shifting leg lameness, anorexia, and/or depression. A history of being exposed to ticks in an endemic area is important.

5.2 Shoulder Region: Growing Dogs

Congenital Shoulder Luxation

Young Small/Large Breed

Congenital shoulder luxation may occur due to deformed or hypoplastic (glenoid dysplasia) glenoid cavity, or developmental laxity of the joint capsule and ligaments.

- Congenital, medial luxation more commonly occurs in small breeds, such as Toy Poodles and Shetland Sheepdogs.
- Lameness usually appears when the animal is young.

History
- Degree of lameness may vary.
- Some small dogs with chronic medial luxation show only mild intermittent lameness.

Physical Examination
- Shoulder manipulation may not cause pain.
- If the glenoid cavity is deformed, reduction of the humeral head may be impossible.

Diagnostic Imaging
- Lateral and ventrodorsal radiographs of the shoulder are evaluated to confirm the diagnosis (Figure 5.2).

Osteochondrosis Dissecans

Young Large Breed

Osteochondrosis dissecans (OCD) commonly occurs in the shoulders, elbows, stifles, and hocks of immature large- and giant-breed dogs; it is rarely reported in small-breed dogs.

- Despite unilateral lameness, this condition is often bilateral.
- A cartilage flap is found on the dorsocaudal humeral head.
- The osteochondral flap may completely detach from the underlying bone and become lodged in the caudoventral joint pouch or bicipital bursa.
- Risk factors for OCD include age, sex, breed (genetic), rapid growth, and nutrient excesses (primarily calcium).
- Degenerative joint disease (DJD) is often the final outcome.
- Clinical signs often develop between 4 and 8 months of age; however, some dogs may not be presented for veterinary evaluation until they are mature or middle-aged.

History
- Affected animals are usually seen with unilateral forelimb lameness.

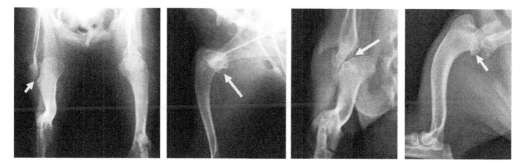

Figure 5.2 Radiographic indications of congenital shoulder luxation (arrows).

- Owners typically report a gradual onset of lameness that improves after rest and worsens after exercise.
- Owners may occasionally associate the onset of lameness with trauma.

Physical Examination

- The shoulder should be palpated and moved through a complete range of motion.
- Affected animals usually show pain when the shoulder is moved into extreme extension (i.e., moving the humerus forward with one hand while the other hand is positioned as a fulcrum on the cranial aspect of the shoulder).

- Extreme flexion of the shoulder may also cause pain.

Diagnostic Imaging

- Diagnosis of OCD is based on radiographic findings evident on lateral projections of the scapulohumeral joints (Figure 5.3); craniocaudal projections do not contribute to the diagnosis, but they may help identify the location of a joint mouse. Arthroscopy may be necessary to confirm a diagnosis of OCD (Figure 5.4).
- Both shoulders should be imaged, because this condition is often bilateral despite unilateral lameness.

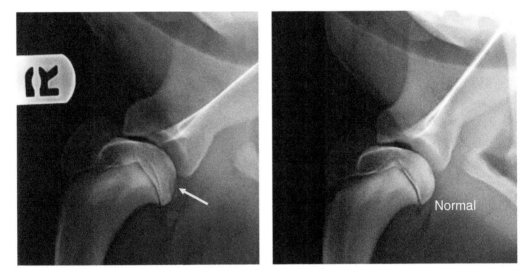

Figure 5.3 Radiographic indications of shoulder OCD (arrow).

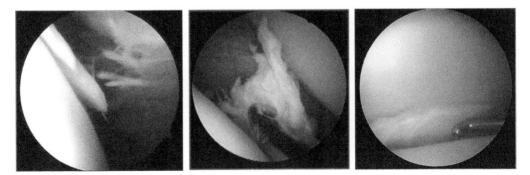

Figure 5.4 Arthroscopic indications of shoulder OCD.

- Multiple views made while the humerus is rotated (pronated and supinated) may be necessary to locate the lesion.
- The earliest radiographic sign of OCD is flattening of the subchondral bone of the caudal humeral head.
- As the disease progresses, a saucer-shaped radiolucent area in the caudal humeral head may be visualized.
- Calcification of the flap may allow visualization of the flap in situ or in the joint if it has detached from the underlying bone (Figure 5.5).
- In chronic cases, large calcified joint mice are often observed in the caudoventral joint pouch or along bicipital bursa.
- Computed tomography (CT) or ultrasound has also been shown to be effective in the diagnosis of OCD of the shoulder (Figure 5.6).

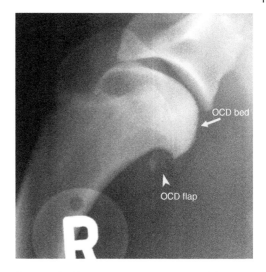

Figure 5.5 Radiographic indications of OCD bed (arrow) and free OCD flap (arrowhead).

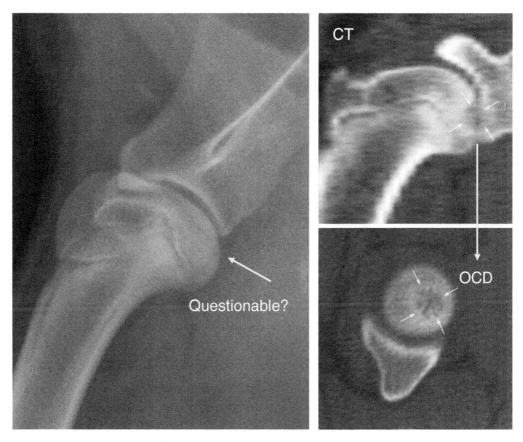

Figure 5.6 Radiographic and CT indications of shoulder OCD (arrows).

5.3 Shoulder Region: Mature Dogs

Shoulder Luxation in Small-Breed Dogs

Adult Small Breed

Traumatic luxation may occur in any age or breed of dog; however, shoulder luxation occurs without a major trauma in small and miniature dog breeds, such as Toy Poodles.

- The scapulohumeral joint is supported by the joint capsule, glenohumeral ligaments, and surrounding tendons (supraspinatus, infraspinatus, teres minor, and subscapularis).

History
- With luxation, affected animals may be non-weight bearing, and the limb is often carried in a flexed position.

Physical Examination
- With medial luxation, the foot is rotated externally and the greater tubercle is palpated medial to its normal location.
- With lateral luxation, the foot is rotated internally, and the greater tubercle is palpable lateral to its normal position.
- Pain and crepitation are evident with shoulder manipulation.

Diagnostic Imaging
- Lateral and ventrodorsal radiographs of the shoulder are evaluated to confirm the diagnosis (Figure 5.7).

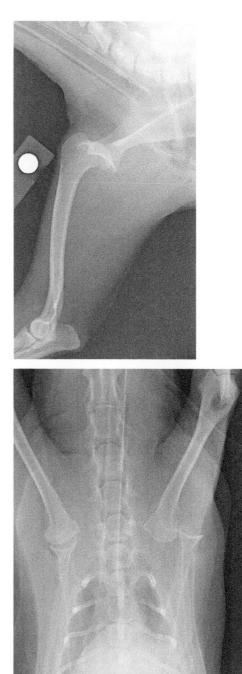

Figure 5.7 Radiographic indications of shoulder luxation.

Shoulder Instability (Shoulder Sprain)

Adult Small/Large Breed

Shoulder instability is characterized by a pathologic increase of the range of motion of the shoulder joint, most commonly in the mediolateral plane. Definitive diagnosis of shoulder instability is made by arthroscopy (Figure 5.8).

- Shoulder instability is due to tearing or stretching of the medial or lateral supportive structures of the shoulder joint.
- The injury may be due to low-grade chronic trauma or acute blunt trauma, resulting in instability and subluxation of the joint without complete luxation.
- Damaged structures may include the medial or lateral glenohumeral ligaments and subscapularis tendon.

History

- This disease occurs most commonly in active dogs, but it may be diagnosed in older animals after years of exercise and activity.

- The animal typically has a history of moderate chronic lameness.

Physical Examination

- A moderate weight-bearing lameness is usually observed on gait analysis.
- Palpation of the limb may demonstrate increased angles of abduction in cases of medial shoulder instability.
- Most dogs have pain on manipulation of the shoulder joint.

Diagnostic Imaging

- Radiographs are usually normal in shoulder instability, although some cases may have enlarged joint space.

Arthroscopy

- Arthroscopic findings may include tearing or laxity of the medial glenohumeral ligament, lateral glenohumeral ligament, or subscapularis tendon.
- Tearing or inflammation of the biceps tendon may also be evident.

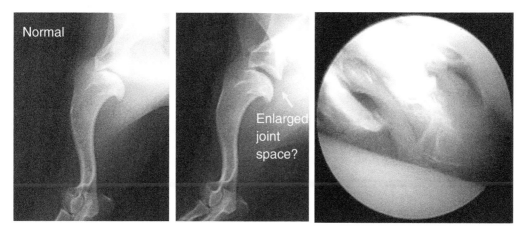

Figure 5.8 Radiographic indications of shoulder instability (arrow) and arthroscopic indications of damaged medial glenohumeral ligament and subscapularis tendon.

Biceps Tendinopathy

Adult Large Breed

Biceps tendon disease (tendinopathy, tendinitis) is a general term that incorporates various types of injury, including tearing of the tendon and inflammation of the tendon and surrounding synovial sheath. Bicipital tenosynovitis is an inflammation of the biceps brachii tendon and its surrounding synovial sheath. Supraspinatus tendinopathy refers to disease of the insertional tendon of the supraspinatus complex that lies craniolateral to the biceps tendon.

- The cause of bicipital tenosynovitis is either direct or indirect trauma to the bicipital tendon, or generalized inflammation (such as OCD).
- Repetitive injury or overuse may be an inciting factor.
- The tendon may be partly or completely ruptured.
- Osteophytes may form in the intertubercular groove.
- The biceps tendon is a significant stabilizer of the shoulder joint, and biceps tenosynovitis may occur in conjunction with generalized shoulder instability (see the earlier shoulder instability section).
- Dogs of any size and age may be affected; working, active dogs are most commonly affected.

History
- Intermittent or progressive forelimb lameness that worsens after exercise is common.
- Tenosynovitis usually presents as a chronic progressive lameness.
- Tearing of the tendon may be associated with an acute onset of lameness.

Physical Examination Findings
- Lameness of one forelimb is usually evident.
- The animal typically stands on the limb but is lame during gaiting.
- Pain may be evident during palpation of the bicipital tendon, especially with concurrent flexion of the shoulder and extension of the elbow.
- Pain may also be evident during palpation of the biceps muscle while the dog is standing.
- Atrophy of the supraspinatus and infraspinatus muscles may be palpable.

Diagnostic Imaging
Radiographic views should include standard lateral projections of both shoulders (Figure 5.9).

- A craniocaudal projection of the humerus (skyline) with the shoulder flexed can be used to identify the bicipital groove.
- Osteophytes in the intertubercular groove may be evident, which should be differentiated from supraspinatus tendinopathy with mineralization (see later section).

Ultrasound provides excellent imaging of the biceps tendon, adjacent tendons, and the bursa and groove.

- Both transverse and longitudinal views should be obtained. The normal biceps tendon has an echogenic linear echo texture in a uniform pattern.
- Acute trauma results in fiber pattern disruption and fluid accumulation within or around the tendon.
- Chronic trauma may demonstrate dystrophic mineralization.
- Fluid accumulation and synovial proliferation of the tendon sheath are easily appreciated, but they cannot be differentiated between those caused by bicipital disease

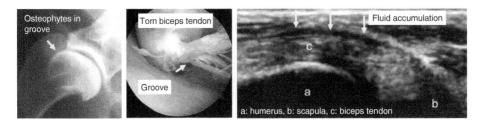

Figure 5.9 Radiographic, arthroscopic, and ultrasonic indications of biceps tendon rupture and tenosynovitis.

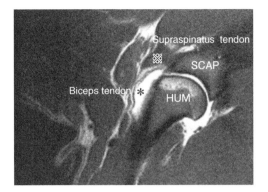

Figure 5.10 MRI representation of shoulder joint with biceps tendinopathy (asterisk). ※ indicates normal fibrocratilage area. HUM, humerus; SCAP, scapula.

and those associated with shoulder joint inflammation of other causes.

Magnetic resonance imaging (MRI) provides excellent imaging of the biceps tendon and all the soft tissue structures surrounding the shoulder joint, and can differentiate inflammation and partial and complete tears of these structures (Figure 5.10).

Supraspinatus Tendinopathy (Mineralization/Calcification)

Adult Large Breed

Supraspinatus tendinopathy refers to mineralized or nonmineralized disease of the insertional tendon of the supraspinatus complex.

- The cause of mineralization of the supraspinatus tendon is unknown, but it may be associated with aging, overuse, trauma, or hypoxia secondary to hypovascularity of the supraspinatus tendon.

- Mineralization may also be associated with tearing of tendon fibers.
- Disease of the biceps and the supraspinatus may occur together.
- Radiographic mineralization is a common incidental finding and is not associated with clinical lameness; therefore, accurate determination of the cause of the lameness is critical.
- Athletic large-breed dogs are affected most commonly.

History
- Lameness may be mild or severe, depending on the severity of the lesion.
- Most animals have a chronic history of lameness.

Physical Examination
- Palpation on the medial aspect of the greater tubercle may cause pain.
- This response may be magnified by shoulder flexion.

Diagnostic Imaging
- With radiography, mineralization within the supraspinatus tendon may be seen adjacent to the greater tubercle using a skyline view.
- The most common ultrasound finding in dogs with supraspinatus tendinopathy is enlargement of the tendon of insertion; MRI may demonstrate enlargement and increased signal in the area of insertion of the supraspinatus tendon (Figure 5.11). Caution: all of these findings can be normal, and therefore accurate determination of the cause of the lameness is vital to creating an appropriate treatment plan.

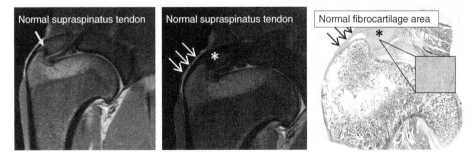

Figure 5.11 MRI and histologic representation of normal supraspinatus tendon (arrows). Asterisk indicates normal fibrocartilage area.

Infraspinatus Contracture

Adult Large Breed

The cause of infraspinatus contracture is unknown, but it appears to be a primary muscle disorder rather than a neurologic or immune-mediated disorder.

- Fibrotic contracture causes muscle contracture and external rotation and abduction of the limb.
- Infraspinatus muscle contracture occurs most often in adult hunting dogs (Figure 5.12).

History
- Acute lameness after strenuous activity in the three weeks before evaluation for infraspinatus muscle contracture is typical.

Physical Examination
- Animals with infraspinatus muscle contracture initially have weight-bearing unilateral forelimb lameness.
- The characteristic gait abnormality occurs secondary to progressive fibrosis and contracture of the infraspinatus muscle.
- As the muscle shortens from contracture, external rotation of the shoulder causes elbow abduction and outward rotation of the paw.

Diagnostic Imaging
- Ultrasonography helps evaluate stabilizers of the shoulder joint.

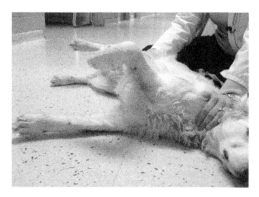

Figure 5.12 Abduction of thoracic limb (inability to adduct) due to infaspinatus contracture.

Osteosarcoma

Adult Large Breed

Osteosarcoma is the most common tumor of the axial skeleton commonly seen in large- and giant-breed dogs.

- Common sites include distal aspect of the radius, proximal aspect of the humerus, distal aspect of the femur, proximal and distal aspect of the tibia, and distal aspect of or diaphyseal region of the ulna.
- The median age is 7 years; however, a small, early peak is seen in dogs 18–24 months of age.
- Large size is a greater determinant of risk: Greyhounds, Rottweilers, and Great Danes may be at increased risk.

History
- Lameness and/or localized limb swelling.
- Pathologic fracture may cause acute, severe lameness.
- Pain, reluctance to walk, and visible swelling.
- Clinical signs may be acute or chronic and progressive.

Physical Examination
- The limb may be enlarged and firm.
- Severe lameness and pain on bone palpation.
- Systemic signs of illness (e.g., fever, anorexia, weight loss) are uncommon in acute stages of the disease.

Diagnostic Imaging
- Radiographic changes are characterized by cortical and trabecular bone lysis, periosteal bone proliferation, and soft tissue swelling (Figure 5.13).
- Thoracic radiographs for evidence of tumor metastasis (CT is more sensitive than radiography).
- Ultimately, histopathology is necessary for confirmation.

Laboratory Findings
Fine-needle aspiration and cytology may be suggestive of bone neoplasia in a large percentage of cases.

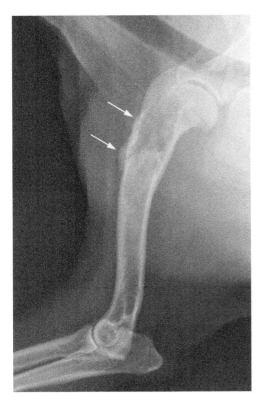

Figure 5.13 Radiographic indications of osteosarcoma (arrows).

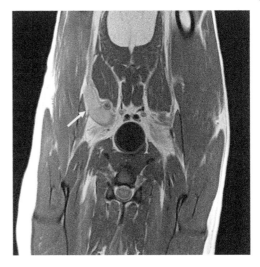

Figure 5.14 MRI indication of peripheral nerve sheath tumor (arrow).

Osteoarthritis

Shoulder OA is less common compared to elbow OA. Radiographs may show osteophytes (Figure 5.15).

- Ultrasound guidance may aid in identifying areas of bone lysis, enabling easier aspiration.
- Cytology of fine-needle aspirates may provide adequate evidence of primary bone tumor to allow initiation of treatment; however, definitive diagnosis of bone neoplasia usually necessitates histologic evaluation of samples obtained by biopsy or excision.

Brachial Plexus Tumor (Peripheral Nerve Sheath Tumor)

Peripheral nerve sheath tumor may involve the peripheral nerves of the brachial plexus (Dewey & da Costa 2015) (Figure 5.14).

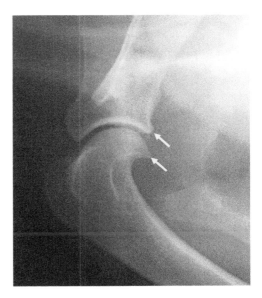

Figure 5.15 Radiographic indications of shoulder OA showing osteophytes (arrows).

5.4 Elbow Region and Antebrachium: Growing Dogs

Condylar Fractures

Young Small/Large Breed

Fractures of the distal humeral condyle (elbow) are common, particularly in young dogs.

- Fractures of the lateral portion of the condyle are frequently diagnosed in young, toy-breed dogs that fall or jump from furniture or the owner's arms with the elbow extended.
- The fracture line passes between the lateral and medial portions of the condyle, crosses the physis, and exits through the metaphysis. Because the physis is involved, the fracture is classified as a Salter IV fracture (Figure 5.16).
- Careful evaluation of the craniocaudal radiograph is essential, because minimal displacement of the intercondylar fracture can occur.

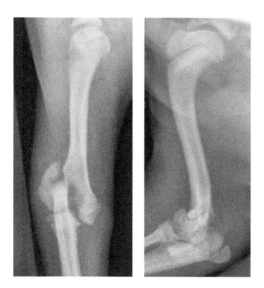

Figure 5.16 Radiographic indications of fracture of lateral part of humeral condyle.

Congenital Elbow Luxation

Young Small/Large Breed

The etiology of congenital elbow luxation is unknown.

- Hypoplasia of the collateral ligament and joint capsule may be related.
- Caudolateral luxation of the radial head is called type I congenital elbow luxation (Figure 5.17).
- Rotation and lateral luxation of the olecranon is called type 2 congenital elbow luxation (Figure 5.18).

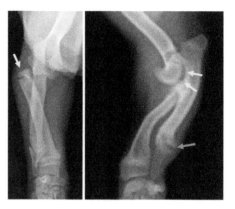

Figure 5.17 Radiographic indications of type I congenital elbow luxation (yellow arrows) and premature physeal closure (blue arrow).

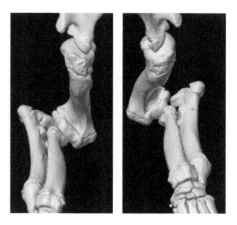

Figure 5.18 CT indications of type II congenital elbow luxation.

Signalment

- Small breeds of dogs are commonly affected: Pugs, Yorkshire terriers, Boston Terriers, Miniature Poodles, Pomeranians, Chihuahuas, Cocker Spaniels, and English Bulldogs are overrepresented.
- The condition can be unilateral or bilateral and is usually recognized when the puppy begins to walk at 3–6 weeks of age.

History

- The history describes the dog's inability to extend one or both front legs and difficulty walking because of the crouching position.
- Smaller dogs tolerate the deformity better and in some cases show minimal or no gait abnormality or pain.

Physical Examination

- Puppies with this condition move with the affected forelimb in flexion.
- If the condition is bilateral, the puppy supports weight on the caudomedial aspect of the forelimbs.
- The elbows cannot be extended.
- The condition is not usually painful.

Diagnostic Imaging

- Lateral and craniocaudal radiographs of the elbow show varying degrees of contact between the radius, the ulna and the humerus.
- A CT scan will better define the deformity.

Antebrachial (Radial and Ulnar) Angular Limb Deformities

Young Small/Large Breed

Synchronous growth of the radius and ulna in the dog is essential for the development of a normal forelimb. The radius receives 40% of its length from the proximal physis and 60% from the distal physis, whereas 85% of the ulnar length comes from the distal physis, with the proximal physis contributing only 15%. In most dogs, growth accelerates rapidly during the fourth to sixth months and tapers off in the ninth or tenth month. This period varies depending on the breed of dog (smaller dogs mature faster than larger dogs).

- Premature closure of the physes in the radius or ulna may lead to an angular limb deformity (ALD).
- The cone-shaped distal ulnar physis frequently sustains a Salter–Harris type V crushing injury during forelimb trauma, due to its unique shape, resulting in complete physeal closure.
- Sequelae include shortening of the ulna with procurvatum (cranial bowing), external rotation of the limb, and shortening of the radius with valgus angulation of the carpus.
- Varying amounts of elbow and carpal incongruity can occur (Figure 5.19).
- Symmetric, complete closure of the distal radial physis results in a shortened but straight radius, elbow incongruity, and a varus angulation of the carpus. The most common deformity of the radius is a caudolateral closure of the distal radial physis, resulting in a valgus deformity.

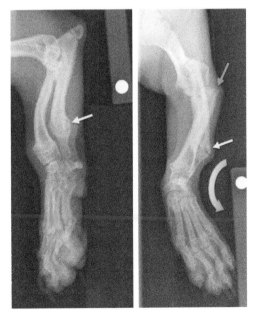

Figure 5.19 Radiographic indications of premature physeal closure (yellow arrows), radial head subluxation (blue arrow), and carpal valgus (curved blue arrow).

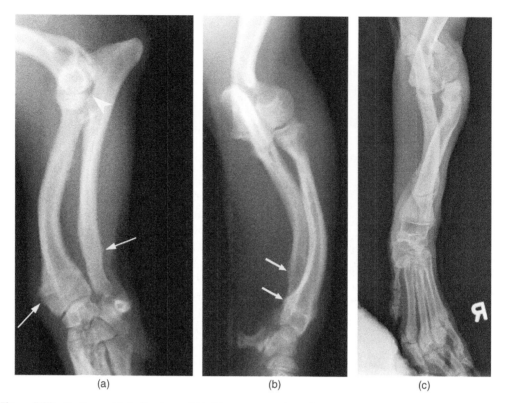

(a)   (b)   (c)

Figure 5.20 Radiographic indications of (a), (b) premature physeal closure (yellow arrows) and elbow (ulnar) subluxation (arrowhead), and (c) radius curvus.

Signalment
Young dogs are affected.

History
- The animal may have a history of fracture of the radius and ulna or an obscure history of trauma.
- This condition can have a genetic predisposition.

Physical Examination
- Dogs with premature closure of the distal ulnar physis show varying degrees of lameness, bowing and shortening of the forelimb, and valgus deviation of the carpus.
- Dogs with symmetric closure of the radial physes may have minimal angular deformity, but may have pain on palpation of the elbow due to the elbow incongruity.

- Dogs with asymmetric closure of the distal radial physis may show an angular deformity depending on the location of the partial closure of the physis.

Diagnostic Imaging
Craniocaudal and lateral radiographs of the affected radius and ulna, which include the elbow and the carpus, are required to assess the deformity.

- The normally functioning physis is radiolucent; a closed physis is seen as bone density.
- Radiographs of the contralateral limb are taken to obtain a control for determining normal radial and ulnar length and normal forelimb anatomy.
- In early cases of premature closure of the distal ulnar physis, a discrepancy in ulnar lengths may be seen before obvious

radiographic signs of physeal closure or fore-limb deformity are noted.

- Always obtain radiographs of the contralateral radius and ulna for comparison. Make length measurements from lateral radiographs.

If torsion of the bone or limb rotation exists, multiple radiographic projections are necessary focusing on the appropriate positioning of each joint (elbow or carpus) (Figure 5.20). However, understanding the extent of the deformity can still quite challenging. Therefore, a CT scan is essential to assess three-dimensional deformities most accurately, including rotational deformities (Figure 5.21).

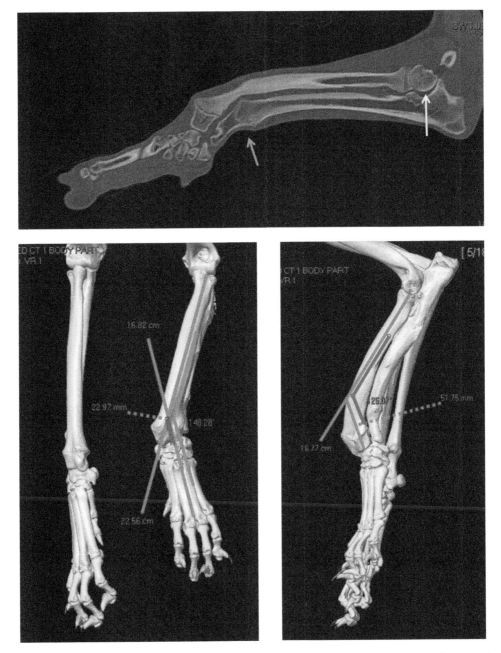

Figure 5.21 CT indications of premature physeal closure (blue arrow), elbow subluxation (yellow arrow), and antebrachial ALD (red and green lines).

Elbow Dysplasia 1

Young Large Breed

Elbow dysplasia likely represents the leading cause of forelimb lameness in the dog (Figure 5.22).

- Several diseases have been designated as components of inherited canine elbow dysplasia. These diseases (e.g., medial coronoid disease, fragmented medial coronoid process [FCP], OCD, ununited anconeal process [UAP], joint incongruity) may differ in terms of pathophysiology, but all are causes of elbow arthrosis.
- Incomplete ossification of humeral condyle (IOHC) is not usually included in the category of elbow dysplasia, although it is a developmental disease that may cause similar clinical signs.
- Selective breeding in Sweden has reduced the prevalence of elbow arthrosis in Rottweilers and Bernese Mountain dogs.

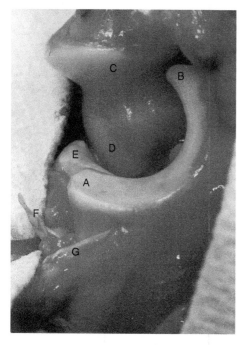

Figure 5.22 Gross anatomy of normal elbow: A, medial coronoid process, B, anconeal process, C, medial part of humeral condyle, D, lateral part of humeral condyle, E, radial head, F, medial collateral ligament, and G, biceps tendon.

Medial Coronoid Disease (Fragmented Medial Coronoid Process)

Medial coronoid disease includes cartilage degeneration, osteonecrosis of the coronoid, fissures within the medial coronoid that may not have led to complete fragmentation, or complete fragment separation from the medial coronoid (Figure 5.23).

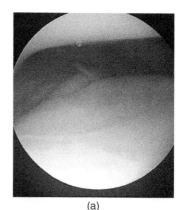

(a)

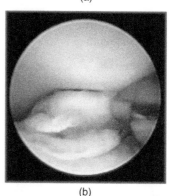

(b)

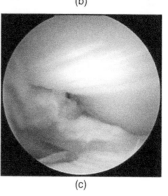

(c)

Figure 5.23 Arthroscopic indications of medial coronoid disease: (a) fissure, (b) displaced fragment, and (c) "kissing lesion."

- FCP is a common type of medial coronoid disease and occurs when a small portion of the medial process of the coronoid separates or detaches from the ulna.
- Medial compartment disease (MCD) often refers to moderate to severe cartilage erosion limited to the medial aspect of the canine elbow joint, and is commonly a consequence of elbow dysplasia, including medial coronoid disease.
- The etiology of medial coronoid disease is unknown.
- Medial coronoid disease may be characterized by complete fragmentation and separation (FCP), partial fissuring of the coronoid, or osteonecrosis. Fissures that develop in the coronoid may or may not progress to fragmentation.
- Developmental elbow incongruity may play a role in the pathophysiology of FCP: trochlear notch dysplasia or malformation, resulting in joint incongruity, may contribute to mechanical overloading and fragmentation of the coronoid.
- FCP may occur secondary to low-grade trauma when a dog lands from a jump (jump-down syndrome).
- The loose coronoid fragment may erode cartilage of the opposing medial part of the humeral condyle ("kissing lesion").

Signalment

Large dogs (Labrador Retrievers, Rottweilers, Bernese Mountain dogs, Newfoundlands, Golden Retrievers, German Shepherds, and Chows) are usually affected.

- The disease process starts when the animal is immature, with clinical signs first becoming apparent at 5–7 months of age. However, dogs may be brought in at any age for OA secondary to FCP and elbow dysplasia.

History

- Forelimb lameness that worsens after exercise may be acute or chronic.

- Owners frequently complain that the dog is stiff in the morning or after rest.

Physical Examination

- Lameness of one forelimb is usually evident.
- Palpation of the dog standing may demonstrate asymmetric joint effusion and periarticular soft tissue swelling.
- Pain on hyperextension of the elbow joint and direct palpation over the medial coronoid area may be the earliest signs of medial coronoid disease.
- Decreased ability to flex the elbow is indicative of more severe OA.
- It is important that the shoulder not be inadvertently flexed and extended during elbow manipulation to prevent mistaking shoulder pain for elbow pain.

Diagnostic Imaging

In many cases, a diagnosis of early medial coronoid disease and FCP may be difficult with radiographs.

- Radiographic views should include a standard lateral of the elbow (Figure 5.24), flexed lateral to expose the anconeal process (Figure 5.25), and a standard craniocaudal view (Figure 5.26).
- Radiographs of both elbows should be taken, because bilateral disease is common.
- Visible fragments are rarely seen.
- The earliest radiographic sign may be "blunting of the medial coronoid process" or small osteophytosis at the joint capsular attachment site on the caudal-proximal aspect of the anconeal process on a flexed lateral view (Figure 5.25).
- The early radiographic sign includes sclerosis of the distal aspect of the trochlear notch (Figure 5.24); this is visible as a loss of the fine trabecular pattern and an increase in opacity.
- Later, a diagnosis of medial coronoid disease and FCP is made on the basis of radiographic signs of DJD; osteophytes associated with the coronoid process and the anconeal process may be visible (Figures 5.24–5.26).

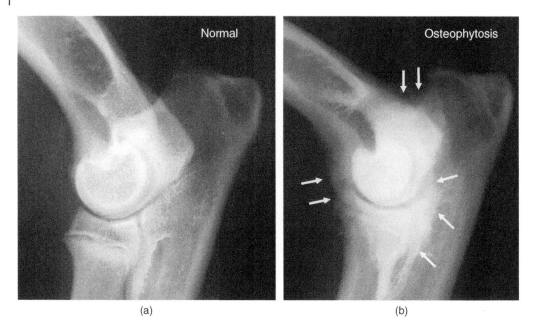

Figure 5.24 (a) Normal elbow. (b) Radiographic indications of elbow dysplasia with increased radio-opacity (osteophytosis) (arrows).

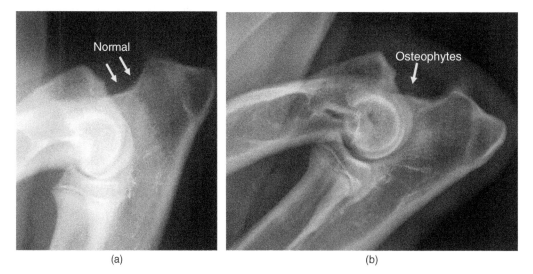

Figure 5.25 (a) Normal anconeal process (arrows). (b) Radiographic indications of elbow dysplasia with osteophytes (arrow).

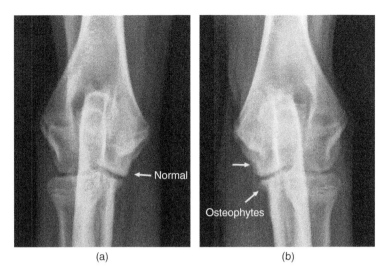

Figure 5.26 (a) Normal elbow showing smooth medial margin (arrow). (b) Radiographic indications of elbow dysplasia with osteophytes (arrows).

- Joint incongruence may be evaluated on radiographs, but evidence suggests a high rate of false positives and false negatives.

CT is helpful for identifying medial coronoid disease and FCP.

- CT scans are more accurate for identifying FCP than survey radiographs.
- CT cannot, however, diagnose superficial fissuring and microcracks of the coronoid.
- CT has the advantage over arthroscopy of being able to diagnose incomplete fragmentation of the medial coronoid that does not reach the cartilage surface.
- CT may aid in evaluating the elbow joint for incongruence or the concomitant occurrence of other forms of elbow dysplasia.

Arthroscopy is the most valuable tool for diagnosing medial coronoid disease and FCP (Figure 5.23).

- Unlike other modalities, arthroscopy enables direct visualization and assessment of the cartilage surface.
- Synovial proliferation is a nonspecific finding that is indicative of elbow joint pathology.

Elbow Dysplasia 2: Osteochondritis Dissecans of the Distal Humeral Condyle

Young Large Breed

Osteochondrosis is a disturbance in endochondral ossification that leads to retention of cartilage; it occurs commonly in the shoulder, elbow, stifle, and hock of immature large dogs. OCD occurs when fissure formation in the abnormal cartilage leads to development of a flap of cartilage and causes clinical signs.

- DJD (osteoarthritis) of the elbow is the final outcome.
- With elbow OCD, a flap covering a defect in the trochlear ridge of the medial part of humeral condyle usually is seen.
- Cartilage erosion at the opposing joint cartilage of the medial coronoid process ("kissing lesion") is different from OCD.

Signalment
- Affected dogs are usually large (Labrador Retrievers, Golden Retrievers).
- The usual age of onset of lameness is 5–7 months.

History
- Forelimb lameness that worsens after exercise may be acute or chronic.

Physical Examination
- Lameness of one forelimb is usually evident.
- Pain may be elicited on elbow extension and on lateral rotation of the forearm.
- A decrease in the animal's ability to flex the elbow is indicative of secondary osteoarthritis. Crepitation during elbow flexion and extension, joint effusion, and periarticular swelling may be noted if OA is present.

Diagnostic Imaging
Radiographic views should include a standard lateral view of the elbow, a flexed lateral view to expose the anconeal process, and a craniocaudal view (Figure 5.27). Radiographs of both elbows should be taken, because bilateral disease is common.

- Definitive radiographic diagnosis of OCD is made when a radiolucent concavity is observed on the distal aspect of the medial part of humeral condyle.
- This lesion is most often identified on the craniocaudal view.
- Radiographic signs of secondary OA are similar to those seen with FCP.

CT Scan
CT scan can be more sensitive than radiographs in identifying an OCD lesion, and again can be helpful for identifying other forms of elbow dysplasia in the same elbow.

Arthroscopy
Arthroscopy permits confirmation of the diagnosis of elbow OCD.

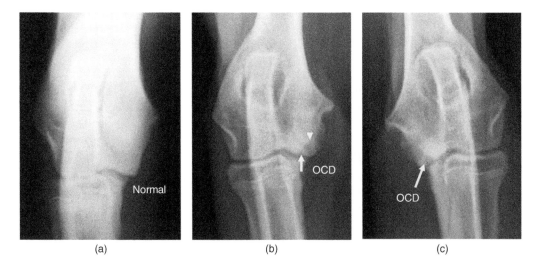

| (a) | (b) | (c) |

Figure 5.27 (a) Normal elbow. (b) Radiographic indications of elbow OCD showing radiolucency (arrowhead) and articular surface defect (arrow). (c) Contralateral elbow of (b): radiographic indications of elbow OCD showing radiolucency and articular surface defect (arrow).

Elbow Dysplasia 3: Ununited Anconeal Process

Young Large Breed

UAP is a disease of large growing dogs in which the anconeal process does not form a bony union with the proximal ulnar metaphysis.

- The anconeal process arises as a secondary center of ossification in the elbow at 11–12 weeks of age.
- It does not fuse to the ulna until 4–5 months of age; therefore, the diagnosis of UAP cannot be made before that age.
- Developmental joint incongruity has been theorized to cause increased pressure or trauma to the anconeal process. The stress of weight bearing on this abnormal cartilage may cause failure of ulnar unification.
- The UAP may be free within the joint, but in most cases it is attached to the ulna with fibrous tissue.
- Ununited or fractured anconeal processes are unstable and result in secondary DJD.
- Concurrent FCP can occur.

Signalment

- German Shepherds are overrepresented.
- The usual age of presentation is 6–12 months; however, some older animals may be seen for lameness caused by secondary OA.

- ALD and elbow incongruity may cause UAP in chondrodystrophic breeds (such as Basset Hounds).

History

- The history is generally intermittent lameness of one or both forelimbs that worsens after exercise.
- Owners frequently complain that the dog is stiff in the morning or after rest.

Physical Examination

Lameness of one forelimb is usually evident.

- Joint effusion and periarticular soft tissue swelling may be palpable.
- The animal may experience pain during joint manipulation, particularly during palpation over the anconeal process.

Diagnostic Imaging

- Radiographic views include a standard lateral view of the elbow, a flexed lateral view to expose the anconeal process, and a craniocaudal view of the elbow made while the elbow is flexed (Figures 5.28 and 5.29).
- Radiographs of both elbows should be taken, because bilateral disease occurs in 20–35% of cases.
- UAP is visible as a lucent, indistinct line separating the anconeal process from the ulna. It is best visualized on the flexed lateral view.

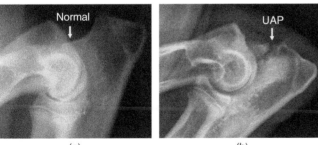

(a)   (b)

Figure 5.28 (a) Normal elbow. (b) Radiographic indications of UAP with secondary arthritic changes (arrow).

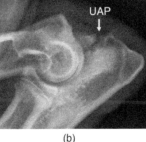

(a)   (b)

Figure 5.29 (a) Radiographic and (b) arthroscopic indications of UAP showing elbow incongruity (asterisk) and articular cracking at the base of UAP (arrows).

Elbow Incongruity (Subluxation)

Young Small/Large Breed

Elbow incongruity (subluxation) may be associated with asynchronous radial or ulnar growth caused by premature closure of one of the distal physes or genetic predisposition (chondrodystrophic breeds).

- The asynchronous growth results in incongruity of the elbow joint because either the radius or ulna is inappropriately short.
- When the ulna is too short, the anconeal process impinges on the humeral trochlea; In some dogs, this may be associated with a UAP.
- When the radius is too short, the radial head is pulled distally and does not articulate with the humeral capitulum.
- The trochlea of the humerus then rests directly on the coronoid process of the ulna.
- This condition is often associated with elbow dysplasia and ALD.

Signalment

- This condition occurs in immature dogs.
- Any breed of dog can be affected; however, Basset Hounds and other chondrodystrophic dogs are more frequently affected with asynchronous growth of the radius and ulna that is not attributable to trauma.

History

- Affected animals often have a history of intermittent lameness.

Physical Examination

- Affected dogs show varying degrees of lameness.
- Pain, crepitation, joint effusion, and limited range of motion may be present during elbow manipulation.

Diagnostic Imaging

- Incongruence of the joint may be investigated with either plain film radiography or CT scan. In severe cases, radio-ulna incongruity is recognized on a lateral or a craniocaudal view of the elbow.
- Routine radiography using standard medial-lateral positioning has been reported to be an inaccurate means of diagnosis of mild incongruity; however, incongruence may be more accurately evaluated on flexed lateral views.
- CT is a more accurate means of evaluating incongruence.
- Arthroscopy has been reported to be an accurate means of diagnosing incongruity.

5.5 Elbow Region: Mature Dogs

Elbow OA

Adult Large Breed

Elbow OA is a common cause of thoracic limb lameness in dogs and is usually a consequence of elbow dysplasia and incongruency (Figures 5.30 and 5.31). Secondary OA may also occur in response to trauma such as elbow fractures or other recognizable joint disease such as IOHC.

Medial Compartment Disease

MCD refers to moderate to severe cartilage erosion limited to the medial aspect of the canine elbow joint. The regions commonly affected include the medial portion of the coronoid process, medial distal aspect of the humeral condyle, and in some cases the medial-most portion of the radial head.

- The etiology of MCD is unknown; however, the most likely cause is mechanical overload or incongruity of the elbow joint (such as medial coronoid disease in elbow dysplasia).
- MCD may be identified with or without concurrent FCP.
- MCD is often the end-stage form of elbow dysplasia, where the inside part of the joint collapses, with eventual grinding of bone on bone.
- Interestingly and importantly, the larger lateral part of the elbow joint appears normal in the vast majority of patients.

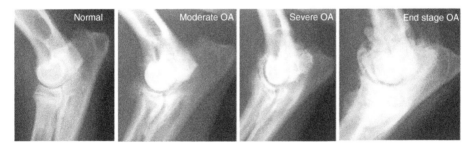

Figure 5.30 Radiographic representation of progression of elbow OA.

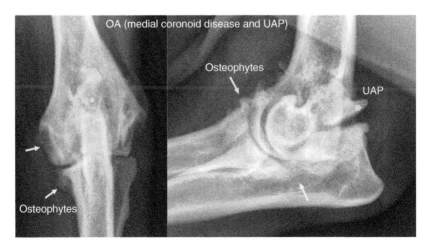

Figure 5.31 Radiographic indications of elbow OA secondary to medial coronoid disease and UAP (asterisk) showing osteophytosis at multiple locations (arrows).

Signalment

- Large-breed dogs are usually affected, although MCD may be diagnosed in any size of dog.

History

- Forelimb lameness that worsens after exercise may be acute or chronic.
- Owners frequently complain that the dog is stiff in the morning or after rest.

Physical Examination Findings

- Lameness of one or both forelimbs is usually evident.
- The gait may appear stiff or stilted if bilateral lameness is present, because the animal may walk with shortened steps.
- Joint effusion and periarticular soft tissue swelling or lateral osteophytosis may be palpable and are most easily felt while the dog is standing.
- Palpation of the elbows should include an evaluation of range of motion. Decreased ability to flex the elbow is indicative of moderate to severe OA.
- Manipulation of the joint is often painful.

Diagnostic Imaging

- In many cases, diagnosis of MCD is suspected on the basis of radiographic signs of DJD (OA).
- Radiographic findings are variable, and severe cartilage damage may be present with minimal radiographic changes.
- Osteophytes associated with the coronoid process and the caudal-proximal anconeal process may be visible. In some cases, severe diffuse osteophytosis may be observed.
- The severity of radiographic changes does not correlate with the severity of cartilage damage.

Arthroscopy

- Arthroscopy is the most definitive tool for diagnosing MCD (Figures 5.32 and 5.33).

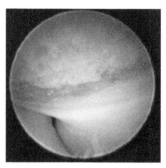

Figure 5.32 Arthroscopic indications of elbow OA showing full-thickness cartilage erosion over the entire medial aspect of the humeral condyle (MCD), with a relatively normal lateral aspect.

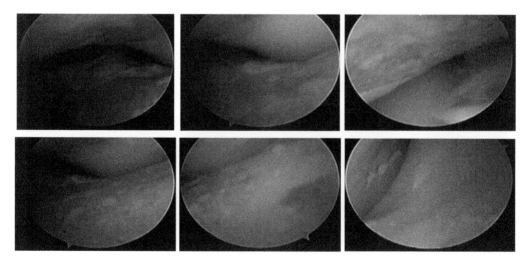

Figure 5.33 Arthroscopic indications of elbow OA showing full-thickness cartilage erosion over the entire medial aspect of the humeral condyle, ulnar notch, and radial head (MCD).

Condylar Fractures

Adult Small/Large Breed

Condylar fractures include fractures of the lateral or medial portions of the condyle, or both, known as a T fracture or Y fracture of the condyle.

- Lateral condylar fractures predominate over medial condylar fractures.

Incomplete Ossification of Humeral Condyle/Humeral Intercondylar Fissure

Adult dogs can sustain lateral condylar fractures due to a minor trauma. In some breeds, particularly Spaniels, incomplete ossification between the medial and lateral portions of the condyle predisposes to condylar fracture and may cause forelimb lameness.

- Normal ossification of the humeral condyle is complete between 8 and 12 weeks.
- The overrepresentation of spaniel breeds suggests a genetic cause.
- The incidence of bilateral disease is reportedly approximately 90%.

Signalment

- Any breed of dog may be affected, but spaniel breeds are overrepresented.
- The age of presentation varies from young to middle-aged dogs, although there is an increased incidence in middle-aged male dogs.

History

- Dogs present with a history of weight-bearing lameness that is worse after exercise; IOHC may lead to a lateral humeral condylar fracture, in which case the patient will present with a non-weight-bearing lameness.
- Dogs with humeral condylar fractures that are possibly the result of IOHC (Spaniel breeds) should have the contralateral limb radiographed to evaluate for contralateral IOHC.

Physical Examination

- Lameness of one forelimb is usually evident.
- Pain can be elicited during elbow joint manipulation.

Diagnostic Imaging

- IOHC may be detected on a craniocaudal view of the elbow joint; however, CT is more sensitive than radiography in the detection of IOHC.
- Sclerosis of the lateral epicondylar crest may be seen radiographically.
- In addition to the area of incomplete ossification, new bone formation may be seen on the lateral humeral epicondyle.

Arthroscopy

- Arthroscopic examination of elbows with IOHC reveals a fissure line in the cartilage at the center of the humeral condyle.

Elbow Luxation

Adult Small/Large Breed

Elbow luxation (or dislocated elbow) is usually associated with blunt trauma of the elbow joint, causing lateral displacement of the radius and ulna with respect to the humerus.

Signalment

- Any age or breed of dog may be affected, although traumatic elbow luxation is rare in immature dogs as they tend to have physeal fractures rather than joint luxation.

History

- The history usually includes trauma, such as a vehicular or dogfight encounter.
- The dog show usually acute non-weight-bearing lameness on the affected limb.

Physical Examination

- Affected dogs are unable to bear weight on the affected limb, and the elbow is carried in a flexed position.
- The forelimb is abducted and externally rotated.
- Palpation of the elbow reveals a prominent radial head, indistinct lateral humeral condyle, and lateral displacement of the olecranon.
- Most animals are in pain and resist elbow extension.

Diagnostic Imaging

- Lateral displacement of the radius and ulna is apparent on a craniocaudal view of the elbow. The lateral view shows an uneven joint space between the humeral condyle and the radius and ulna.
- Avulsion fractures of the medial or lateral condyle of the humerus may be evident.
- Because of the traumatic cause, thoracic radiographs before surgery are indicated.

5.6 Carpal Region and Distal Limb: Growing Dogs

Fractures in Small-Breed Dogs

Young Small Breed

Toy-breed dogs are often brought in after apparently minimal trauma of jumping or falling.

- The fracture site is commonly the distal diaphyseal region (Figure 5.34). Physeal fracture can occur, but is less common compared with distal diaphyseal fractures.
- Affected animals usually have non-weight-bearing lameness after trauma.

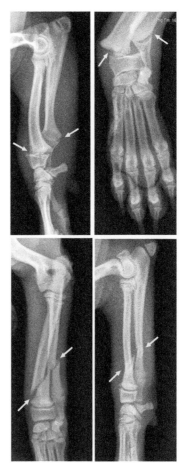

Figure 5.34 Radiographical indications of physeal and diaphyseal fractures (arrows).

Puppy Carpal Laxity Syndrome

Young Small/Large Breed

Carpal laxity syndrome is hyperextension of the carpus in young growing dogs.

- Carpal laxity syndrome is thought to be due to malnutrition, poor footing, and improper exercise in young puppies.
- The result is weakness and irregular tension between the extensor and flexor muscle groups and secondary carpal laxity.
- Young puppies (6–8 weeks old) of any breed may be affected.
- Orthopedic examination demonstrates carpal and in some cases tarsal laxity and a palmigrade stance.
- There is no significant swelling or pain of the joints.
- Radiographs of the joints are normal.

Hypertrophic Osteodystrophy

Young Large Breed

Hypertrophic osteodystrophy (HOD) is a disease that causes disruption of metaphyseal trabeculae in the long bones of young, rapidly growing dogs. The cause of HOD is unknown.

Signalment

- This disease affects young, rapidly growing, large-breed dogs, and males are affected more often than females.
- Clinical signs are usually first noted at 3–4 months of age; however, they may occur as early as 2 months.
- Relapses may occur as late as 8 months of age.
- Weimaraners may be at increased risk.

History

- An acute onset of lameness is often reported, and puppies may be so severely affected that they refuse to walk.
- Inappetence and lethargy are commonly reported by owners.

Physical Examination

- Findings on physical examination range from mild lameness to severe lameness affecting all four limbs.
- More severely affected animals are often unable to stand or walk.
- Long bone metaphyses are swollen, warm, and painful on palpation.
- Swelling is often present in all four limbs; however, forelimb swelling may be more obvious, especially in distal radial metaphyses.
- Severely affected dogs may be depressed, anorexic, and pyrexic.

Diagnostic Imaging

- Radiographs of affected long bones reveal an irregular radiolucent zone in the metaphysis, parallel and proximal to the physis (Figure 5.35).
- This gives the appearance of a "double physeal line."
- Metaphyseal flaring with increased bone opacity occurs because of periosteal proliferation in later stages of the disease.

Laboratory Findings

- Bacteremia has rarely been reported in association with HOD.

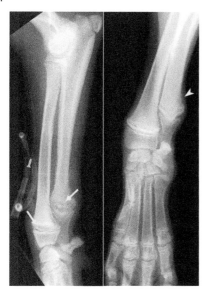

Figure 5.35 Radiographic indications of HOD (arrows) and periosteal reaction (arrowhead).

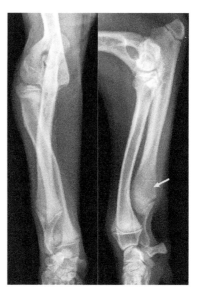

Figure 5.36 Radiographic indications of distal ulnar physeal injury (arrow).

Distal Ulnar Physeal Injury/Premature Physeal Closure/Angular Limb Deformity

Young Large Breed

The cartilaginous physis is weaker than surrounding bone and ligaments, making it more susceptible to injury. Trauma resulting in compression of the zone of proliferating cells and destruction of the chondrocytes causes premature physeal closure. This often results from trauma to the V-shaped distal ulnar physis in dogs.

- ALD is a common sequela of this injury (see Section 5.4).
- Ulnar physeal fractures occur in immature dogs with open physes.
- Fractures in this area are not visible radiographically until 2–3 weeks after trauma, when premature closure of the physis is observed (Figures 5.36 and 5.37).

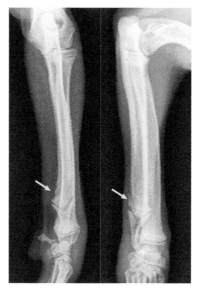

Figure 5.37 Radiographic indications of distal ulnar physeal injury and periosteal reaction (arrows).

Retained Cartilaginous Cores

Young Large (Giant) Breed

Retained cartilaginous cores (in distal ulna) may represent failure of the growth plate cartilage to convert to metaphyseal bone.

- This condition predominantly affects large to giant immature dogs.
- It is associated with ulna shortening and ALD (Figure 5.38).

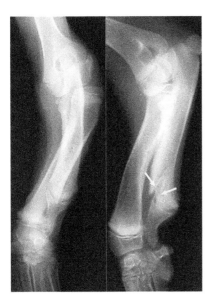

Figure 5.38 Radiographic indications of retained cartilaginous core in distal ulnar physis (arrows), and associated antebrachial ALD and elbow subluxation.

5.7 Carpal Region and Distal Limb: Mature Dogs

Radial/Ulnar Fractures

Adult Small Breed

Toy-breed dogs often fracture the radius and ulna after apparently minimal trauma of jumping or falling (Figure 5.39).

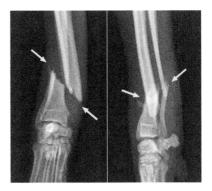

Figure 5.39 Radiographic indications of radius/ulna distal diaphyseal fractures (arrows).

Neoplasia: Osteosarcoma

Adult Large Breed

Osteosarcoma is the most common tumor of the axial skeleton commonly seen in large- and giant-breed dogs. Common sites include the distal aspect of the radius, proximal aspect of the humerus, distal aspect of the femur, proximal and distal aspect of the tibia, and distal aspect of or diaphyseal region of the ulna (Figure 5.40).

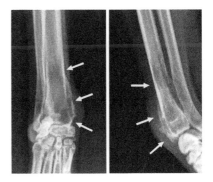

Figure 5.40 Radiographic indications of osteosarcoma in distal radius (arrows).

Immune-Mediated Poly-arthropathy

Adult Small/Large Breed

Idiopathic nonerosive inflammatory arthropathies (IMPA) have no identifiable cause and are diagnosed by ruling out all other causes of polyarthritis.

- Radiographs of affected joints usually reveal either no abnormalities or synovial fluid effusion and periarticular soft tissue swelling (Figure 5.41).

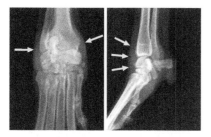

Figure 5.41 Radiographic indications of joint swelling (arrows), associated with cytologic diagnosis of IMPA.

Erosive IMPA (Rheumatoid Arthritis)

Rheumatoid arthritis is an erosive, noninfectious, inflammatory joint disease characterized by chronic, bilaterally symmetric, erosive destruction of the joints.

- Radiographs of the joints show a generalized loss of mineralization, radiolucent foci, and irregular joint margins (Figure 5.42).
- Bone proliferation may also be present. Soft tissue swelling and joint effusion may be evident.

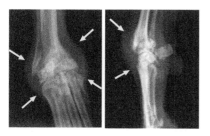

Figure 5.42 Radiographic indications of joint swelling (arrows) and erosive changes in periarticular structures, associated with cytologic diagnosis of IMPA.

Hypertrophic Osteopathy

Adult Small/Large Breed

Hypertrophic osteopathy (HO) is a diffuse periosteal reaction resulting in new bone formation around the metacarpal, metatarsal, and long bones.

- HO can affect all four limbs.
- It can be a paraneoplastic syndrome (such as primary and metastatic lung tumors), or it may be associated with other diseases (e.g., granulomatous lesions, chronic megaesophagus, patent ductus arteriosus, bacterial endocarditis, heartworm disease).
- The precise pathophysiology of this disease is unknown.

Signalment
- Any breed or size of dog may be affected; however, because it is most commonly associated with neoplasia, HO is usually seen in older animals.

History
- Dogs are usually brought in because of lethargy, reluctance to move, and swelling of the distal extremities.

Physical Examination
- Affected limbs are warm and swollen.
- Because this condition occurs secondary to diseases elsewhere in the body, an effort should be made to identify the underlying causative factors.

Diagnostic Imaging
- Radiographs of the limbs reveal a periosteal proliferation (Figure 5.43).

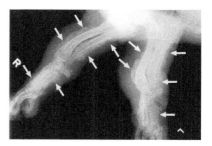

Figure 5.43 Radiographic indications of HO showing periosteal reaction at multiple locations (arrows).

- Thoracic radiographs and an abdominal ultrasound should be performed to identify underlying abdominal disease. Advanced imaging modalities (CT, MRI) may be necessary in some cases to identify the primary lesion.

Carpal Hyperextension

Adult Small/Large Breed

Carpal hyperextension results from a jump-down-type trauma causing loss of palmar fibrocartilage support and weight-bearing function.

- Polyarthritis (such as IMPA) may lead to severe soft tissue damage with progressive collapse of the joint to a palmigrade stance, which needs to be differentiated from carpal hyperextension injury.

Signalment

- Any age or breed and either sex of dog or cat may be affected with traumatic hyperextension.

History

- Acutely affected animals usually have a non-weight-bearing lameness.
- Most animals return to using the leg within a week, but they are lame and have a plantigrade stance.

Physical Examination

- Acute injuries show clear indications of swelling, pain, and instability.
- There is mild to moderate pain on manipulation of the joints.

Diagnostic Imaging

- Standard craniocaudal and medial-to-lateral radiographs are needed to detect bone fractures or joint malalignment associated with complete luxation of the joints; however, stress radiographs should be performed to assess carpal integrity accurately and identify the joint level of the hyperextension injury (Figure 5.44).
- With the patient under heavy sedation or general anesthesia, it should be positioned in lateral recumbency with stress applied to the foot to place the carpus in maximum extension.
- A medial-to-lateral radiograph is produced with the carpus in maximal extension.
- If the contralateral limb is normal, similar images may be taken for comparison.

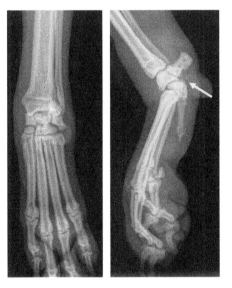

Figure 5.44 Radiographic indications of carpal hyperextension with abnormal joint angle (arrow).

Carpal Collateral Ligament Injury (Instability, Subluxation)

Adult Small/Large Breed

Carpal instability (subluxation) may result from loss of collateral ligamentous support (sprain) of the antebrachial carpal joint.

- Carpal collateral ligament injuries are usually due to trauma.
- Either the medial or lateral collateral ligament may be involved.
- Most injuries involve the radiocarpal joint.

Signalment

- Any age or breed and either sex of dog or cat may be affected.

History

- Acutely affected animals usually have a non-weight-bearing lameness.

Physical Examination

- Acute injuries show clear indications of swelling, pain, and instability.
- Palpation of the carpus demonstrates the ability to "break open" the joint either medially or laterally.

Diagnostic Imaging

- Standard craniocaudal and medial-to-lateral radiographs are needed to detect bone fractures or joint malalignment associated with complete luxation of the joints. However, stress radiographs should be performed to assess carpal integrity accurately and identify the level of the collateral ligament injury.
- Integrity of the collateral ligaments is determined by obtaining craniocaudal views of the carpus while a medial and lateral stress is applied to the foot (Figure 5.45).

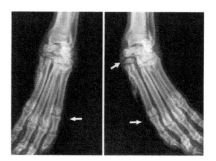

Figure 5.45 Radiographic indications of carpal medial collateral injury (yellow arrow) with "stress view" radiographs (white arrows).

Abductor Pollicis Longus Tendinopathy (Stenosing Tenosynovitis)

Adult Large Breed

Stenosing tenosynovitis of the abductor pollicis longus muscle can cause chronic thoracic limb lameness in mid-sized to large breed dogs.

- A firm swelling at the medial aspect of the antebrachiocarpal joint may be noted.
- Flexion and rotation of the carpus may cause pain.
- Radiographs of the carpus are characterized by soft tissue swelling, and irregular mineralization located medial to the radial sulcus with varying mineralization (Figure 5.46).

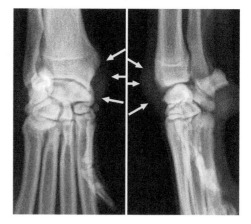

Figure 5.46 Radiographic indications of swelling due to abductor pollicis longus tendinopathy (arrows).

Fractures in Distal Limb

Any Size

Metacarpal and metatarsal bone fractures are common in dogs.

- Metacarpal and metatarsal fractures are classified according to location (e.g., base or proximal end of the bone, shaft, or diaphysis; head or distal end of the bone) (Figure 5.47).
- Luxations of the metacarpophalangeal joints or interphalangeal joints typically occur in working dogs or racing greyhounds.

Sesamoid Pathology

Two palmar or plantar sesamoid bones are present per metacarpophalangeal or metatarsophalangeal joint, numbered one through eight beginning on the medial side (Figure 5.48).

- Sesamoid fractures occur after excessive tension on the digital flexor tendons; sesamoid bones 2–7 of the forelimb are most often affected.

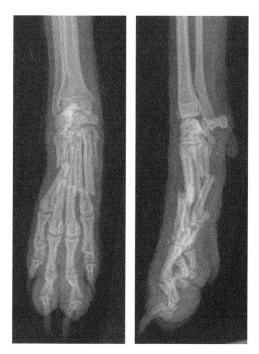

Figure 5.47 Radiographic indications of metacarpal fractures (arrows).

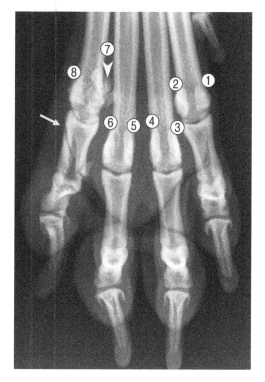

Figure 5.48 Radiographic indications of 7th sesamoid fracture (arrowhead) and proximal phalangeal fracture (arrow).

Carpal/Metacarpal OA

Adult Large Breed

Carpal and metacarpal OA (Figure 5.49) is less common compared to elbow OA.

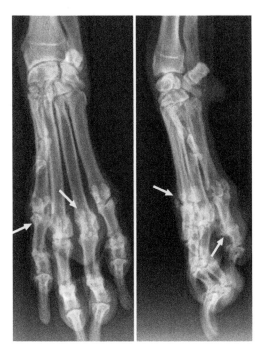

Figure 5.49   Radiographic indications of arthritic changes in metacarpal and phalangeal joints (arrows).

Digit Conditions

Adult Large Breed

Digit pathologies include neoplasia, chronic bacterial or fungal infections, osteomyelitis, or severe trauma.

- Affected digits are swollen and painful with thickened, dystrophic, or absent claws.
- Squamous cell carcinoma is the most common tumor identified in canine digits (Figure 5.50); however, numerous neoplastic processes can occur in this location (such as malignant melanomas, soft tissue sarcomas, osteosarcomas, and mast cell tumors).
- Digital tumors occur in older dogs (mean age 10 years) and are often initially misdiagnosed as infections.
- They occur most often in male large- to medium-breed dogs (10 to >30 kg).
- Clinical signs include lameness, digit swelling and ulceration, and a fixed protruding, deviated, or lost nail.

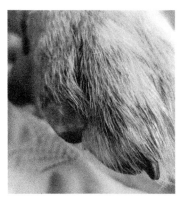

Figure 5.50   Gross appearance of nail-bed tumors (such as squamous cell carcinoma) or infections.

Reference

Dewey, C.W., & da Costa, R.C. (2015). *Practical Guide to Canine and Feline Neurology*, 3rd ed. Chichester: Wiley-Blackwell.

6

Pelvic Limb Conditions

Kimberly A. Agnello

6.1 Common General Conditions

Panosteitis

Young Large Breed

See Chapter 5 (Figures 6.1 and 6.2).

Idiopathic Immune-Mediated Polyarthritis (IMPA)

See Chapter 5.

Erosive IMPA (Rheumatoid Arthritis)

See Chapter 5.

Septic Arthritis

See Chapter 5.

Osteomyelitis

See Chapter 5.

Rickettsial/Anaplasmal/Lyme Poly-Arthropathy

See Chapter 5.

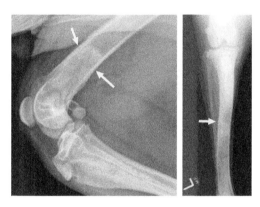

Figure 6.1 Radiographic indications of panosteitis of femur and tibia (arrows).

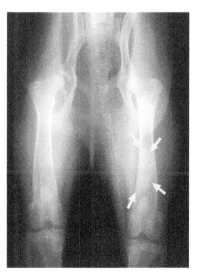

Figure 6.2 Radiographic indications of panosteitis of femur (arrows).

6.2 Hip Region: Growing Dogs

**Femoral Head Necrosis
(Legg–Perthes Disease)**

Young Small Breed

Avascular necrosis of the femoral head is a noninflammatory aseptic necrosis of the femoral head that occurs in young patients before closure of the capital femoral physis.

- Femoral head necrosis results in collapse of the femoral epiphysis because of an interruption of blood flow.
- The reason for the loss of blood flow is not known for certain; however, an autosomal recessive gene has been proposed as a genetic cause.
- The bone substance is weakened mechanically during the revascularization period, and normal physiologic weight-bearing forces may cause collapse and fragmentation of the femoral epiphysis.
- Fragmentation (fractures) of the femoral epiphysis and osteoarthrosis cause pain and resulting lameness.

Signalment
- Legg–Perthes disease is diagnosed in young, small-breed dogs (i.e., <10 kg).
- The peak incidence of onset is 6–7 months with a range of 3–13 months, and males and females are equally affected.
- This condition is usually unilateral and occurs bilaterally in approximately 10% of affected dogs.

History
- Affected animals are usually presented for evaluation of a slow-onset, weight-bearing lameness that worsens over a 6–8-week period.
- Lameness may progress to non-weight bearing.
- Some clients report an acute onset of clinical lameness; in these patients, sudden collapse of the epiphysis may cause acute exacerbation of an already present but imperceptible lameness.

Physical Examination
- Manipulation of the hip joint consistently elicits pain in affected animals.
- Limited range of motion, muscle atrophy, and crepitus may be present with advanced disease.

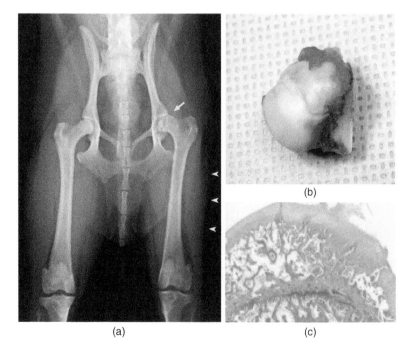

(a)   (b)   (c)

Figure 6.3 (a) Radiographic indications of femoral head necrosis (arrow) and associated muscle atrophy (arrowheads). (b) Gross appearance and (c) histologic representation of its pathology.

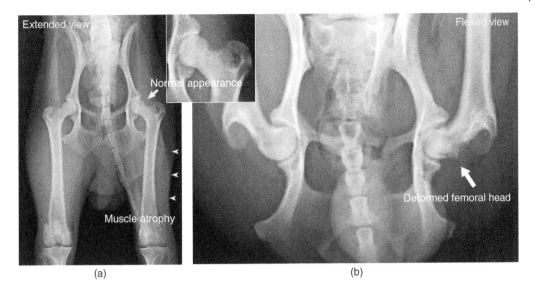

(a)   (b)

Figure 6.4 (a) Radiographic representation of normal-looking femoral head (arrow) and associated muscle atrophy (arrowheads) in a standard extended view. (b) Radiographic indications of femoral head necrosis showing deformed femoral head (white arrow) in a flexed ("frog leg") view.

Diagnostic Imaging

- Radiographs may show deformity of the femoral head, shortening and/or lysis of the femoral neck, and foci of decreased bone opacity within the femoral epiphysis (Figures 6.3 and 6.4).

- A flexed hip ("frog leg") view is often useful to detect abnormal shape of the affected femoral head.
- A computed tomography (CT) scan may become necessary to identify lysis or cavitation within an affected femoral head that maintains a relatively normal shape (Figure 6.5).

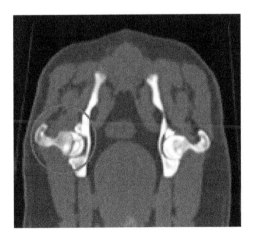

Figure 6.5 CT indications of femoral head necrosis showing deformed femoral head with fissures and cavitation (red circle).

Hip Dysplasia

Young Large Breed

Hip dysplasia is the abnormal development of the coxofemoral joint, characterized by subluxation (laxity) of the femoral head in younger dogs and mild to severe degenerative joint disease (DJD) in older dogs.

- The causes of hip dysplasia are multifactorial. Both hereditary and environmental factors play a part in the development of abnormal bone and soft tissue; however, hereditary factors are the primary determining factors.
- Subluxation stretches the fibrous joint capsule, causing pain and lameness.
- Acetabular cancellous bone is easily deformed by continual dorsal subluxation of the femoral head.
- Physiologic responses to joint laxity (subluxation) are proliferative fibroplasia of the joint capsule and increased trabecular bone thickness.
- These changes relieve pain associated with capsular sprain and trabecular fractures; however, the surface area of articulation is still reduced, leading to premature wear of articular cartilage, exposure of subchondral pain fibers, and lameness.

Signalment

- The incidence of hip dysplasia is highest in large-breed dogs.
- History and clinical signs vary with the patient's age.
- Two populations of dogs are usually presented: juvenile patients with hip laxity and mature patients with osteoarthritis (OA).

History

- Symptoms in young patients include difficulty rising after rest, exercise intolerance, and intermittent or continual lameness.
- As animals mature they may develop additional signs attributable to hip joint pain.
- Progressive DJD in these patients results in difficulty rising, exercise intolerance, lameness after exercise, atrophy of the pelvic musculature, and/or a waddling gait (stiff short-stride gait) attributed to abnormal movement of the rear limbs.
- Patients are often seen for evaluation of lameness that has suddenly worsened during or after increased activity or injury.

Physical Examination

- In juvenile patients with lameness (5–10 months of age), physical findings include pain during extension, external rotation, and abduction of the hip joint, and poorly developed pelvic musculature.
- Hip examination performed under general anesthesia shows increased laxity of the hip joints, as evidenced by abnormal angles of reduction and subluxation.
- Many juvenile dogs spontaneously improve with increasing age after conservative management. This is due to elimination of subluxation by scar tissue formation around the joint.
- Physical examination findings in older animals include pain during hip joint extension, reduced range of motion, and atrophy of pelvic musculature.
- There is generally no detectable joint laxity because of the proliferative fibrous response, but crepitus may be detected on joint manipulation.
- It is important to note that clinical signs do not always correlate with radiographic findings.

Diagnostic Imaging

- The standard radiographic view for diagnosis of hip dysplasia is the ventrodorsal view of the pelvis, with rear limbs extended symmetrically and rotated inward to center the patellae over the trochlear grooves (Figure 6.6).

- The dog must be heavily sedated or anesthetized for proper relaxation and positioning.
- CT or arthroscopy will provide more detailed information.

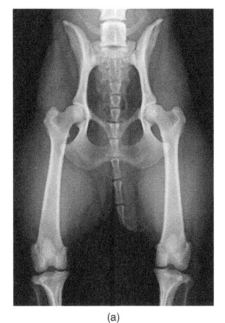

(a)

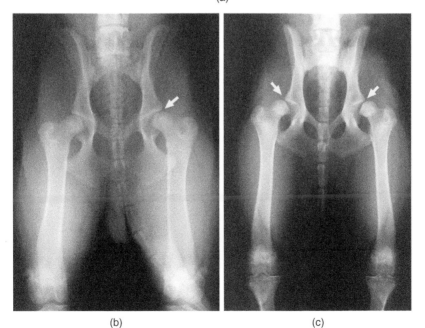

(b)   (c)

Figure 6.6 (a) Normal hip. (b, c) Radiographic indications of hip dysplasia showing subluxation of the femoral head (arrows).

Femoral Capital Physeal Fracture

Young Small/Large Breed

Physeal fractures involve the growth plates in immature animals. The capital physis is the proximal femoral physis of the femoral head.

- Capital physeal injuries may occur without significant trauma.
- Proximal physeal fractures are generally Salter I or Salter II fractures.
- The capital physis functions to provide femoral neck length until the animal is approximately 8 months of age.

Signalment

- Most affected animals are younger than 10 months.

History

- Most animals are presented for evaluation of acute non-weight-bearing lameness.
- Minor trauma such as a fall may be sufficient to separate the growth plate.

Physical Examination

- Animals with proximal physeal fractures usually exhibit non-weight-bearing lameness with pain and crepitation on manipulation of the hip joint.
- Some animals are weight bearing and do not have detectable crepitus referable to the hip joint. These animals usually have minimal displacement of the femoral head.

Diagnostic Imaging

- Standard ventrodorsal and mediolateral projections of the femur are required to confirm the diagnosis. Some animals may require sedation.
- A fractured capital physis with minimal displacement may be difficult to detect using an extended limb ventrodorsal radiographic projection.
- A ventrodorsal view with the limbs in "frog leg" position may help confirm the diagnosis in such cases (Figure 6.7).

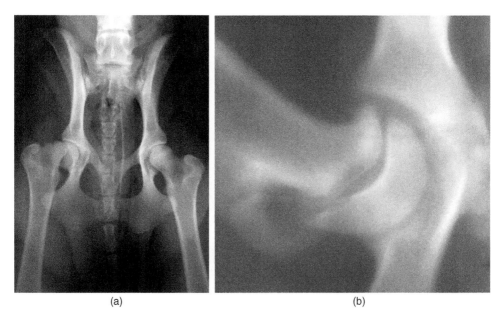

(a)   (b)

Figure 6.7 Radiographic indications of femoral capital physeal fracture in (a) a standard extended view and (b) a flexed ("frog leg") magnified view.

6.3   Hip (and Pelvic) Region: Mature Dogs

Hip (Coxofemoral) Luxation

Adult Small/Large Breed

Hip luxation is a traumatic displacement of the femoral head from the acetabulum.

- Hip luxation typically results in craniodorsal displacement of the femoral head relative to the acetabulum.
- Affected animals usually show a unilateral non-weight-bearing lameness.
- When the femur is displaced craniodorsally, the limb is carried adducted, with the stifle externally rotated.
- When it is displaced caudoventrally, the limb is carried abducted, with the stifle internally rotated.

Signalment

- Any age or breed and either sex of dog may be affected.

History

- Hip luxation typically results from trauma. However, it can occur with a minimal trauma in small dogs.

Physical Examination

- Manipulation of the limb causes crepitus or pain.
- A palpable lack of symmetry is noted between the tuber ischii and greater trochanter on the affected side compared with the normal limb.

Diagnostic Imaging

- Diagnosis of hip luxation should be confirmed with ventrodorsal and lateral radiographs (Figure 6.8).
- Before a treatment method is chosen, radiographs should be carefully evaluated for evidence of avulsion of the fovea capitis, associated hip joint fractures, and degenerative changes secondary to hip dysplasia.

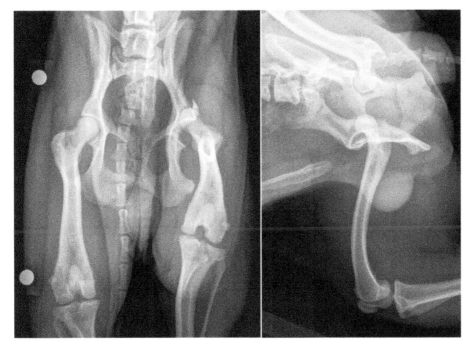

Figure 6.8   Radiographic indications of cranio-dorsal hip luxation with an associated small fracture.

Hip Osteoarthritis (Degenerative Joint Disease)

Adult Large Breed

Hip OA is a is usually a sequela to hip dysplasia and incongruency (Figure 6.9). Secondary OA may also occur in response to trauma such as fractures.

Septic Arthritis

Osteoarthritis is known to increase the risk of septic osteoarthritis in humans and likely increases the risk in dogs.

Diseases such as canine hip dysplasia/DJD may increase the risk of septic arthritis, and this diagnosis should be considered when examining patients with hip pain and severe OA.

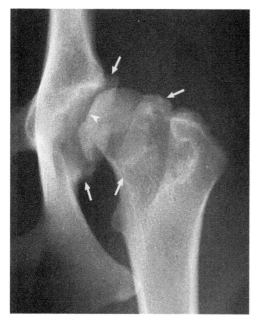

Figure 6.9 Radiographic indications of hip OA with osteophytosis (arrows) and deformed and displaced femoral head (arrowhead).

Lumbosacral Disease (Cauda Equina Syndrome)

Adult Large Breed

The cauda equina is the leash of nerve roots derived from the terminal spinal cord segments from L7 caudally (Cd1–Cd5). The lumbosacral area, or lumbosacral junction, is the bone (e.g., L7 vertebra, sacrum) and connective tissue (e.g., L7–S1 articular facet joint capsules, interarcuate ligament, disc) enclosing the cauda equina (Dewey & da Costa 2015).

- Dogs with cauda equina lesions often appear painful on extension of the hip joints. This may be because the extension is pulling on nerve roots that are already irritated by a disease process at the lumbosacral junction. Alternatively, these patients may have concurrent hip dysplasia/OA that is not of clinical significance, or of lesser clinical significance than the cauda equina disorder.
- Because clinical signs of lumbosacral disease can mimic those of hip dysplasia, it is important not to confuse the two disorders, especially in dogs that are predisposed to both disorders and may have radiologic evidence of hip dysplasia (e.g., German Shepherds).
- In lumbosacral disease, careful palpation of the lumbosacral area is required to elicit a painful response, whereas the patient may appear to be in constant pain with conditions such as discospondylitis and vertebral tumor.

Signalment

- Degenerative lumbosacral disease typically affects adult (usually middle-aged to older) large-breed dogs.
- There is evidence that the presence of lumbosacral transitional vertebrae is a predisposing factor for developing both degenerative lumbosacral stenosis (DLSS) and hip dysplasia.

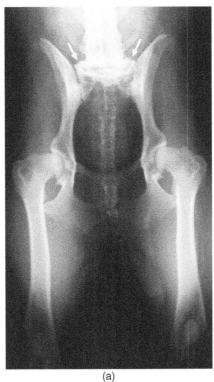

(a)

(b)

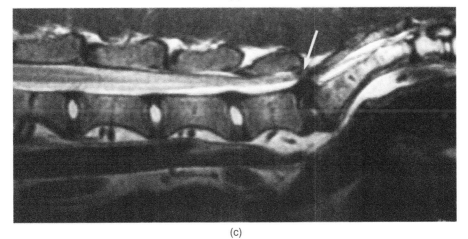

(c)

Figure 6.10   (a, b) Radiographic indications of lumbosacral instability and arthritic changes (arrows) and (c) magnetic resonance imaging (MRI) indications of lumbosacral lesion (arrow).

History

- A unilateral or bilateral pelvic limb lameness, which may be exacerbated by increased activity, may also indicate hyperesthesia in the area of the lumbosacral region and cauda equina.

Physical Examination

- The most common clinical sign associated with lesions of the cauda equina is pain.
- Some patients exhibit obvious discomfort when rising or sitting down. Others may be reluctant to jump or climb stairs.
- Proprioceptive deficits can be as mild as delayed proprioceptive positioning reactions or as severe as pelvic limb ataxia with dragging of the dorsal aspect of the toes (knuckling).

- Dogs with cauda equina lesions are not typically ataxic.
- In some cases, the patient may exhibit an abnormally low tail carriage, which the owner often notices.

Diagnostic Imaging

- MRI is often required for definitive diagnosis (Figure 6.10).

Neoplasia around the Hip Region

Adult Large Breed

The most common primary bone tumor is osteosarcoma, which may affect pelvis and proximal femur (Figure 6.11).

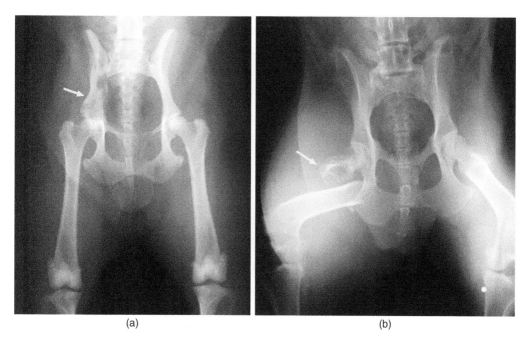

(a) (b)

Figure 6.11 Radiographic indications of (a) pelvic and (b) femoral osteosarcoma (arrows).

6.4   Stifle Region: Growing Dogs

Medial Patellar Luxation

Young Small Breed

Medial patellar luxation (MPL) is a displacement of the patella from the trochlear sulcus. Genu varum is a deformity associated with severe MPL, resulting in a "bow-legged" appearance.

- MPL is a common cause of lameness in small-breed dogs, but it also occurs in large-breed dogs.
- Most patients with patellar luxation have associated musculoskeletal abnormalities, such as medial displacement of the quadriceps muscle group, lateral torsion of the distal femur, a lateral bowing of the distal one-third of the femur, femoral epiphyseal dysplasia, rotational instability of the stifle joint, or tibial deformity.

Signalment

- Dogs of any age or breed and either sex may have MPLs, but small- and toy-breed dogs are most frequently affected.
- MPLs are more common than lateral patellar luxations (LPLs) in large-breed dogs; however, large dogs have a higher percentage of lateral luxations than small dogs.

History

- Most affected animals have an intermittent weight-bearing lameness.
- Owners may report that the dog occasionally holds the leg in a flexed position for one or two steps.
- Dogs with grade IV patellar luxations have severe lameness and gait abnormalities.

Physical Examination

- The diagnosis of MPL is based on finding or eliciting MPL during a physical examination.
- Physical findings vary and depend on the severity of luxation.
- Patients with a *grade 1 luxation* generally show no lameness, and the diagnosis is made as an incidental finding on physical examination.
- Patients with a *grade 2 luxation* show occasional "skipping" when walking or running. These patients occasionally stretch the lateral retinacular structures and develop a non-weight- bearing lameness.
- Lameness in patients with a *grade 3 luxation* varies from an occasional skip to a weight-bearing lameness.
- Patients with a *grade 4 luxation* walk with the rear quarters in a crouched position because they are unable to extend the stifle joints fully. The patella is hypoplastic and may be found displaced medially alongside the femoral condyle.

Diagnostic Imaging

- With a grade 3 or grade 4 luxation, standard craniocaudal and medial-to-lateral radiographs show the patella to be displaced medially, whereas with a grade 1 or grade 2 luxation the patella may be within the trochlear sulcus or may be displaced medially (care must be taken to properly position the limb to eliminate artifactual appearing luxations) (Figures 6.12 and 6.13).
- Full-limb radiographs may show varus or valgus deformities and torsion of the tibia and femur.
- Careful radiographic positioning is critical, as poor positioning results in false-positive limb deformity on radiographs.
- For more severe cases requiring long bone osteotomy and correction, special views (coronal or skyline view of the femur) or CT scan aid in determining the specific type and degree of deformity.

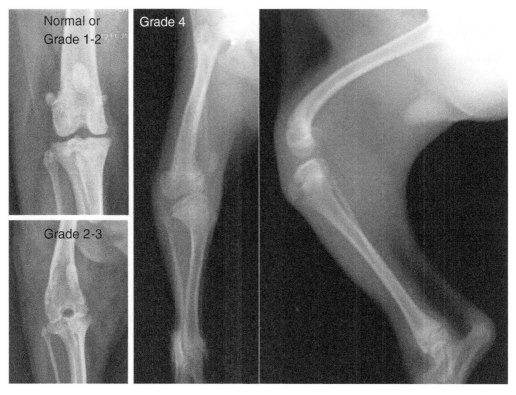

Figure 6.12 Examples of radiographic representations of MPL (grades 1–4).

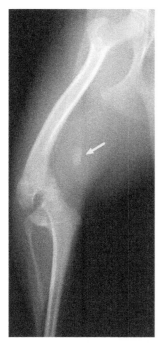

Figure 6.13 Radiographic indications of grade 4 MPL with femoral and tibial deformities and ectopic patella (arrow) in a small dog.

Lateral Patellar Luxation

Young Large Breed

LPL is an intermittent or permanent displacement of the patella from the trochlear sulcus. Genu valgum is a deformity affecting giant-breed dogs associated with LPL, resulting in a "knock-kneed" appearance.

- LPL is seen most often in large-breed dogs, but it does occur in small- and toy-breed dogs.
- The cause is unknown.

Signalment
- Dogs of either sex and any age or breed may be affected.
- LPLs are more frequently seen in large breeds of dogs than in small and toy breeds.

History
- Affected animals are most commonly seen for evaluation of an intermittent, weight-bearing lameness.

Physical Examination

- Physical examination findings vary and depend on the severity of luxation.
- The diagnosis is determined by finding or eliciting lateral luxation of the patella and eliminating other causes of rear-limb lameness.
- Patients with a grade 4 luxation walk with the rear quarters in a crouched position because of inability to extend the stifle joints fully.

Diagnostic Imaging

- With a grade 3 or grade 4 luxation, standard craniocaudal and medial-to-lateral radiographs consistently show the patella to be displaced laterally (Figures 6.14 and 6.15).
- CT scan aids in determining the specific type and degree of deformity.

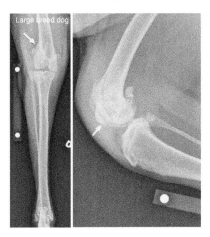

Figure 6.14 Radiographic indications of grade 3 LPL showing displaced patella (arrows) in a large dog.

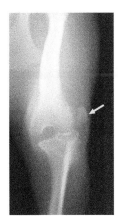

Figure 6.15 Radiographic indications of grade 4 LPL showing ectopic patella (arrow) in a small dog.

Osteochondritis Dissecans of the Stifle

Young Large Breed

Osteochondritis dissecans (OCD) or osteochondrosis is a disturbance in endochondral ossification that leads to retention of cartilage; it occasionally occurs in the stifle of immature large dogs.

- With OCD of the stifle, a piece of cartilage and subchondral bone is usually observed that involves the medial surface of the lateral femoral condyle (most frequently affected) or the medial femoral condyle.
- The condition is often bilateral.

Signalment

- Affected dogs are usually large (e.g., German Shepherds, Great Danes) and young, with the average age at onset of lameness being 5–7 months (range, 3 months–3 years).

History

- Rear-limb lameness, which worsens after exercise, may be acute or chronic and mild or severe.
- Often the onset of the lameness is insidious.
- Owners frequently complain that the dog is stiff in the morning or after rest, and they are generally concerned that the dog may have hip dysplasia.

Physical Examination

- Lameness of one rear limb is usually evident.
- There may be stifle joint effusion and crepitation, especially if DJD is progressing.
- In immature dogs, a slight cranial drawer may be noted, especially with muscle atrophy. However, when the cranial drawer is tested in animals with stifle OCD, drawer motion should stop abruptly, indicating that the cranial cruciate ligament (CCL) is intact (normal).

Diagnostic Imaging

- Radiographic views should include standard craniocaudal and lateral views of the stifle (Figures 6.16 and 6.17).
- Oblique views may be needed to observe the extent of the lesion.
- Radiographs of both stifles should be obtained to identify bilateral disease.

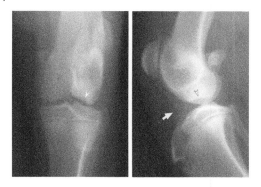

Figure 6.16 Radiographic indications of stifle OCD showing an articular defect (arrowheads) and joint effusion (arrow).

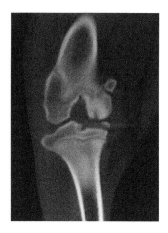

Figure 6.18 CT indications of stifle OCD showing subchondral bone defect and surrounding sclerosis.

- Definitive radiographic diagnosis of OCD is made when a radiolucent concavity is observed on the medial or lateral femoral condyle.
- More subtle radiographic signs include flattening of the articular surface and subchondral sclerosis.
- CT scan and arthroscopy provide definitive diagnosis of OCD (Figure 6.18).

Long Digital Extensor Tendon Avulsion

Young Large Breed

Long digital extensor (LDE) tendon avulsion can occur with a trauma, and needs to be distinguished from stifle OCD (Figure 6.19).

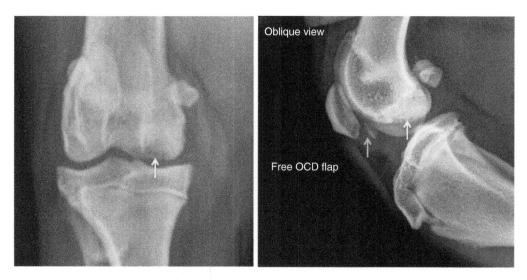

Figure 6.17 Radiographic indications of stifle OCD showing an articular defect ("OCD bed"; yellow arrow) and a free osteochondral "OCD flap" (blue arrow).

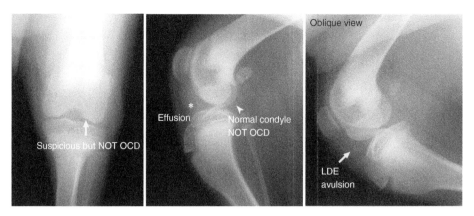

Figure 6.19 Radiographic indications of LDE tendon avulsion showing severe stifle effusion (asterisk), normal femoral condyle (arrowhead), and avulsed origin of LDE (arrow).

Physeal Fractures of the Stifle

Young Small/Large Breed

Physeal fractures involve the growth plates in immature animals.

- Physeal injuries may occur without significant trauma. The cartilaginous physis is weaker than surrounding bone and ligaments, making it more susceptible to injury.
- Distal femoral physeal fractures are generally Salter II physeal fractures.
- Proximal tibial physeal fractures are usually Salter I or II fractures, although rarely Salter III or IV fractures occur. With Salter I or II fractures and concurrent fracture of the fibula, the epiphysis may be displaced caudolateral to the tibial diaphysis, and additional injury to collateral ligaments may occur.

Signalment
- Young dogs are affected.

History
- Most animals are presented for evaluation of acute non-weight-bearing lameness.
- The trauma may or may not have been witnessed by the owner.

Physical Examination
- Animals with physeal fractures present with swelling, pain, and crepitus on manipulation of the stifle region.

Diagnostic Imaging
- Standard craniocaudal or ventrodorsal and mediolateral projections of the femur and tibia are required to confirm the diagnosis (Figure 6.20).
- Additional oblique and skyline projections are useful in evaluating the articular surface of the trochlea and femoral condyles if fissures or fractures of these structures are suspected.

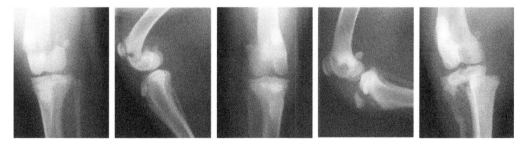

Figure 6.20 Examples of radiographs indicating physeal fractures of distal femur, tibial tuberosity, and proximal tibia.

- Comparison radiographs of the contralateral limb are often beneficial, particularly with tibial tuberosity avulsions.

Metaphyseal Fractures of the Proximal Tibia

Proximal tibial metaphyseal fractures occur in skeletally immature dogs from minimal trauma and commonly have a characteristic curvilinear fracture configuration (Figure 6.21). They affect mainly small-breed dogs, with a predominance for terrier breeds.

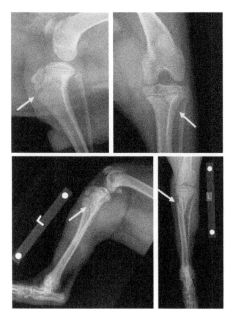

Figure 6.21 Examples of radiographs indicating metaphyseal fractures (arrows) of proximal tibia.

Quadriceps Contracture ("Tie-Down")

Muscle contracture or fibrosis (quadriceps tie-down, fracture disease of the rear limb) may occur when normal muscle–tendon unit architecture is replaced with fibrous tissue, resulting in functional shortening of the muscle or tendon. This shortening may cause abnormal motion in adjacent joints. Myopathy is another term used to describe muscle disease, and this condition can be also called fibrotic myopathy.

- Quadriceps muscle contracture usually occurs after distal femoral fracture in young dogs; however, congenital contracture of the quadriceps muscle has been reported.
- Inadequate fracture stabilization, excessive tissue trauma during surgery, or prolonged limb immobilization with the stifle in extension may singly or in combination contribute to quadriceps contracture.
- It is often associated with Salter–Harris type I or II fracture of the distal femur in puppies.
- Quadriceps contracture may occur after splinting in extension for as little as 5–7 days.
- In later stages, the disease also causes bone atrophy, atrophy of cartilage in the stifle, intraarticular fibrosis, and eventual ankylosis of the stifle joint.
- The cause of congenital quadriceps contracture and the reason why contracture occurs most commonly in young dogs are unknown.

Signalment

- Any age, breed, or sex of dog may develop quadriceps muscle contracture; however, it most commonly occurs in immature patients after distal femoral fracture when inappropriate repair has been done and/or postoperative physical rehabilitation has been inadequate.

History

- Animals with quadriceps muscle contracture are usually evaluated for lameness 3–5 weeks after sustaining femoral trauma.
- Application of an external splint (such as a Schroeder–Thomas splint) for stabilization of a femoral fracture is a common cause.
- The stifle joint of dogs with quadriceps muscle contracture has a limited range of motion.
- Contracture may be such that the stifle joint appears hyperextended.
- Cranial thigh muscles are generally atrophied and palpated as a thickened cord.

Diagnostic Imaging

- Radiographic changes vary depending on the type, severity, and stage of trauma.

6.5   Stifle Region: Mature Dogs

**Cranial Cruciate Ligament Rupture/
Meniscal Syndrome (Cruciate Disease)**

Adult Small/Large Breed

CCL injury (rupture) with a cascade of events that include synovitis, effusion, stifle joint instability, progressive OA, and medial meniscus injury is often called "cruciate disease" (CCLD).

- The CCL functions primarily to limit cranial translation of the tibia relative to the femur.
- The CCL also limits internal rotation of the tibia and the interaction of the cranial and caudal cruciate ligaments during flexion also provides a limited degree of varus–valgus support to the flexed stifle joint.
- CCL failure can result from degenerative and traumatic causes. The categories are interrelated because ligaments weakened by degeneration are more susceptible to trauma.
- With ligament degeneration, even repetitive normal activities can cause progressive rupturing of the ligament.
- In many cases, the underlying pathologic condition is present in both stifles and a high percentage of dogs either have bilateral cruciate ligament rupture, or they rupture the contralateral ligament within 1–2 years.
- Partial rupture of the CCL results in lameness with minimal detectable stifle instability and progressive radiographic signs of OA.
- Partial rupture generally proceeds to complete ligament rupture with time.
- Stifle instability and synovitis result in articular cartilage degeneration, periarticular osteophyte development, and capsular fibrosis.
- The immobile medial meniscus is subject to injury in the unstable joint.

Signalment
- Either sex and any age or breed of dog may be affected.

History
- Clinical presentation can be acute or chronic.
- The dog usually maintains a weight-bearing lameness.
- The owners may report that the dog sits with the affected limb out to the side of the body.
- Lameness is typically worse after exercise or after sleeping.
- Acute worsening of lameness may indicate additional meniscal injury to cruciate disease.
- Partial CCL tears are difficult to diagnose in the early stages of injury. Initially, affected animals have a mild weight-bearing lameness associated with exercise, which will resolve with rest. This stage of the disease may last for many months. As the ligament continues to tear and the stifle becomes increasingly unstable, degenerative changes worsen, and lameness becomes more pronounced and does not resolve with rest.
- Dogs of any age may have bilateral subacute or chronic bilateral CCL rupture. These dogs may have a presumptive neurologic disease because the dog may be unable or unwilling to support weight in either hind limb.

Physical Examination
- Joint effusion may be palpable adjacent to the patellar tendon.
- Pain on hyperextension of the joint is commonly present in dogs with partial tears.
- Instability can be difficult to elicit.
- Patients with chronic tears may have thigh muscle atrophy (compared with the normal limb).
- An enlargement along the medial joint surface (medial buttress) can often be palpated and is caused by osteophyte formation along the trochlear ridges and fibrous tissue formation along the medial condyle and proximal tibia.

Diagnostic Imaging

- Radiographs are helpful in ruling out other causes of stifle joint pain and lameness such as neoplasia around the stifle region (e.g., synovial cell sarcoma).
- Radiographic findings include effusion ("fat pad sign") and osteophyte formation along the trochlear ridge, the caudal surface of the tibial plateau, and the distal pole of the patella (Figures 6.22–6.24).
- Thickening of the medial fibrous joint capsule ("medial buttress") and subchondral sclerosis are also evident in chronic cases.

- Avulsion of the CCL attachment may be seen in young dogs.
- MRI has been used for evaluation of the cruciate ligament in dogs; however, it is not sensitive to detect early changes, and the cost and necessity for general anesthesia limit the use of this technique.

Combination of Cruciate Ligament Rupture and Medial Patellar Luxation

CCL rupture occurs secondary to MPL (Figure 6.25; see Chapter 12).

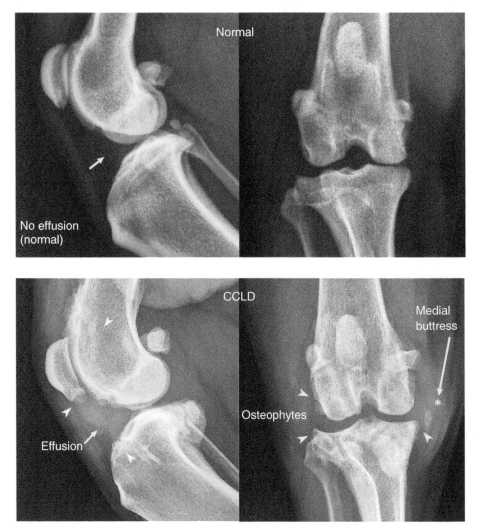

Figure 6.22 Radiographic indications of normal (top) and abnormal stifle (bottom) showing signs of CCLD such as joint effusion (arrow), osteophytes (arrowheads), and periarticular fibrosis (asterisk on medial buttress).

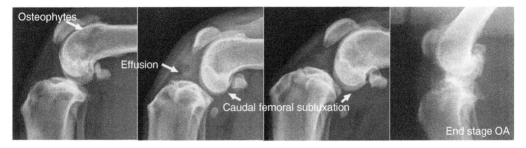

Figure 6.23 Radiographic representation of progression of CCLD and stifle OA.

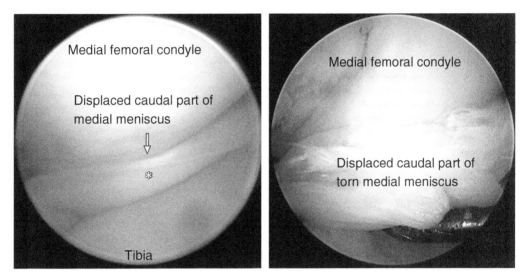

Figure 6.24 Arthroscopic indications of meniscal injury with displacement of caudal part of the medial meniscus (asterisk).

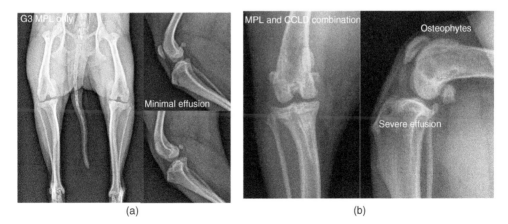

Figure 6.25 (a) Radiographic indications of grade 3 MPL. (b) Radiographic indications of combination of grade 3 MPL and CCLD.

Neoplasia around the Stifle Region

Adult Small/Large Breed

The most common primary bone tumor is osteosarcoma, which commonly affect the distal femur and proximal tibia. The tumors arising from synovial tissue are called synovial sarcomas (malignant synovioma, synovial cell sarcoma), histiocytic sarcomas, and synovial myxomas.

Signalment

- Osteosarcoma and synovial sarcomas occur most commonly in large, middle-aged dogs; however, a breed predisposition has not been identified.
- Greyhounds, Rottweilers, and Great Danes may be at increased risk.
- Bernese Mountain dogs, Flat-Coated Retrievers, and Golden Retrievers may be affected more commonly with histiocytic sarcomas.

History

- Affected dogs are severely lame.
- A mass near a joint may occasionally be noticed by owners.
- Masses may grow slowly for a period; rapid growth may then occur.

Physical Examination

- Masses vary in size, but are usually firm.
- Compression on the mass causes pain.

Diagnostic Imaging

- Radiographs of involved joints are needed to evaluate the extent of bone and soft tissue involvement (Figures 6.26–6.29).

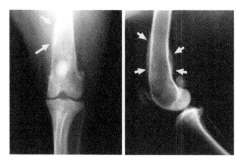

Figure 6.26 Radiographic indications of osteosarcomas (arrows) in distal femur.

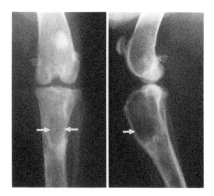

Figure 6.27 Radiographic indications of osteosarcomas (arrows) in proximal tibia.

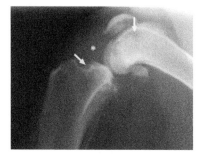

Figure 6.28 Radiographic indications of intraarticular soft tissue opacity due to synovial cell sarcoma (asterisk) with associated bony lysis (arrows).

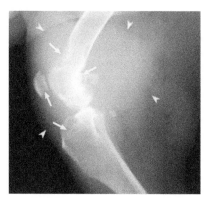

Figure 6.29 Radiographic indications of soft tissue swelling due to synovial cell sarcoma (arrowheads) with associated bony lysis (arrows).

- Bone changes (e.g., lysis of subchondral bone and cortex, new bone production) are often noted.
- Thoracic radiographs or contrast-enhanced CT scans should be performed to evaluate for the presence of pulmonary metastasis.

Gracilis/Semitendinosus Fibrotic Myopathy

Muscle contracture or fibrosis may occur when normal muscle–tendon unit architecture is replaced with fibrous tissue, resulting in functional shortening of the muscle or tendon.

- Gracilis or semitendinosus fibrotic myopathy occurs most often in German Shepherd dogs or Belgian Shepherds.
- Fibrotic myopathy of the iliopsoas and the sartorius muscles has also been reported.
- The cause of fibrotic myopathy is unknown.
- The muscle fibers are replaced with dense fibrous connective tissue, causing a non-painful lameness.

Signalment
- Gracilis or semitendinosus myopathy occurs in young adult, male German Shepherds and in Belgian Shepherds.
- Traumatic gracilis muscle injuries occur in Greyhounds.

History
- A history of insidious onset of rear-limb lameness is characterized by an altered gait associated with gracilis or semitendinosus myopathy.

Physical Examination
- Dogs with gracilis or semitendinosus myopathy have a shortened stride, rapid elastic medial rotation of the paw, external rotation of the hock, and internal rotation of the stifle during the mid to late swing phase of the stride ("circumduction gait").
- The lameness is more pronounced at a trot.
- Affected muscles are palpable as a distinct taut band differentiated by the location of origin.
- Most dogs exhibit a nonpainful lameness.
- Abduction of the hip and extension of the stifle and hock may be limited.

Diagnostic Imaging
- Radiography is not usually helpful in these cases.
- Ultrasound examination is typically used to determine the extent and severity of the abnormality.

Collateral Ligament Injury

The medial and lateral collateral ligaments function in concert to limit varus–valgus motion of the stifle joint.

- Isolated medial or lateral collateral ligament tears are rare in small animals.
- Most injuries that involve the medial or lateral collateral ligaments occur in conjunction with injury to other primary and secondary restraints of the stifle joint.

Signalment
- Any age or breed and either sex of dog may be affected.

History
- This injury may occur while the animal is exercising or during a traumatic incident.

Physical Examination
- Diagnosis of collateral ligament injury is based on palpation.
- It is important to remember that the stifle joint must be extended to examine for collateral injury.
- The valgus stress test is used to evaluate integrity of the medial collateral ligament.
- The varus stress test is used to evaluate integrity of the lateral collateral ligament.

Diagnostic Imaging
- Radiographs should be obtained to determine if bone fragments are associated with ligament damage.
- Stress radiographs are useful for demonstrating an increase in medial or lateral joint space.

6.6 Tarsal Region and Distal Limb: Growing Dogs

Osteochondritis Dissecans of the Tarsus

Young Large Breed

OCD is a disturbance in endochondral ossification that leads to cartilage retention; it occurs in the hocks of immature large-breed dogs.

- With OCD of the talus, a large piece of cartilage and subchondral bone is usually observed involving the medial (most frequently affected) or lateral trochlear ridge.

Signalment
- Affected dogs are usually large; Rottweilers are most frequently affected.
- The average age of onset of lameness is 5–7 months, and the condition affects both males and females.

History
- Rear-limb lameness that worsens after exercise may be acute or chronic.
- Owners frequently report that the dog is stiff in the morning or after rest.

Physical Examination
- Lameness of one rear limb is usually evident.
- Pain may be elicited on hock flexion.
- Joint effusion and periarticular swelling may be noted.

Diagnostic Imaging
- Radiographic views of the tarsus should include a standard lateral view, a flexed lateral view, and a craniocaudal view (with the hock flexed) (Figure 6.30).
- Radiographs of both tarsi should be obtained, because bilateral disease is common.
- Definitive radiographic diagnosis of OCD is made when a radiolucent concavity is observed on the medial or lateral trochlear ridge.
- A CT scan can be used to better evaluate the trochlear ridges if OCD is suspected or if diagnosis cannot be confirmed on survey radiography.

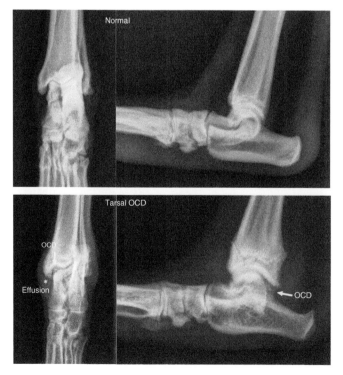

Figure 6.30 Radiographic indications of tarsal OCD (arrow) with associated joint effusion (asterisk).

Tibial and Fibular Physeal Fractures

Young Small/Large Breed

Distal tibial physeal fractures are usually Salter I or II fractures.

Signalment

- These fractures occur in immature dogs with open physes.

History

- Affected animals usually have non-weight-bearing lameness after trauma.
- Owners may be unaware that trauma has occurred.

Physical Examination

- Palpation of the limb may reveal swelling, pain, crepitation, and instability of the adjacent joint.

Diagnostic Imaging

- Craniocaudal and lateral radiographs of the affected tibia and fibula are required to diagnose Salter I to Salter IV fractures (Figure 6.31).
- Comparison radiographs of the opposite limb are often beneficial.

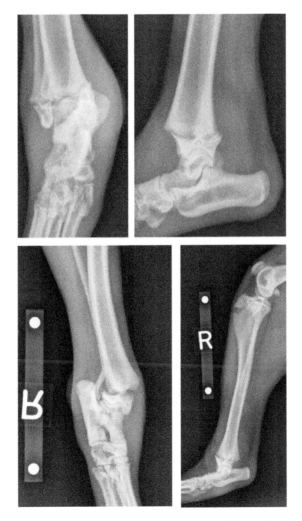

Figure 6.31 Examples of radiographs indicating physeal fractures of distal tibia/fibula.

6.7 Tarsal Region and Distal Limb: Mature Dogs

Common Calcaneal (Achilles') Tendon Pathology

Common calcaneal tendon ruptures are seen most often in sporting and performance athlete breeds; however, any breed may be affected.

- Injury may arise from an acute traumatic episode or from chronic progressive stretching of the tendon.
- The injury may be a partial or complete rupture of the Achilles' tendon.
- Chronic injuries more commonly occur in sporting breeds (e.g., field trial dogs and bird hunting dogs) and are often bilateral.
- Bilateral chronic degeneration of the common calcanean tendons is relatively common in Doberman Pinschers, although the cause is unknown.

Signalment

- Any age, breed, or sex of dog or cat may be affected.
- Athletic dogs are most commonly affected.
- Doberman Pinschers may have idiopathic bilateral common calcanean tendon degeneration.

History

- Affected animals usually exhibit weight-bearing lameness with a "dropped hock" appearance.

Physical Examination

- Postural changes and careful palpation of the muscle–tendon unit can confirm the diagnosis.
- Tarsal hyperflexion is often noted in animals with common calcaneal tendon rupture.
- The patient will be weight bearing but will walk plantigrade because of hyperflexion of the tarsus.

- Patients with chronic tendon injury show varying degrees of tarsal hyperflexion depending on the length of time the injury has been present.
- If the tendon of the superficial flexor muscle is intact, the digits will flex in addition to tarsal hyperflexion.

Diagnostic Imaging

- Standard craniocaudal and medial-to-lateral radiographs are indicated to determine whether bone avulsion is present or not (Figures 6.32 and 6.33).
- Ultrasonography can help determine the location of tendon fiber disruption and may differentiate between partial and complete tears.

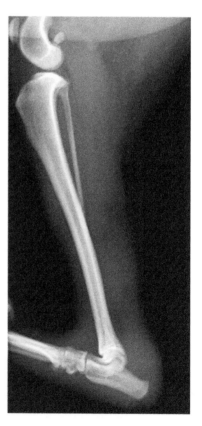

Figure 6.32 Radiographic indications of common calcaneal tendon injury showing discontinuation of the tendon and tarsal hyperflexion.

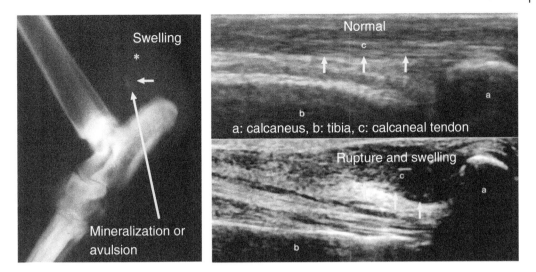

Figure 6.33 Examples of radiographs and ultrasound images indicating common calcaneal tendon injury and associated pathology.

Superficial Digital Flexor Tendon Displacement

Superficial digital flexor tendon displacement (SDFD) occurs when the tendon slides off the calcaneus. The displacement causes lameness of the affected limb.

- The superficial digital flexor tendon is the most superficial part of the common calcaneal tendon and inserts distally on the toes.
- Tearing of the retinaculum that keeps the tendon over the tuber calcanei allows the tendon to displace medially or laterally.
- Lateral displacement is more common than medial displacement.

Signalment
- SDFD is rare in dogs.
- Shelties may be overrepresented for SDFD.
- No age or size predisposition is known.

History
- History may include insidious or acute onset of rear-limb lameness.

Physical Examination
- Dogs with SDFD have hind-limb lameness and swelling of the tip of the calcaneus.
- In most cases, it is possible to feel the tendon slide off the tip of the calcaneus.

Diagnostic Imaging
- Radiography is typically not helpful.
- Ultrasound examination is not necessary for diagnosis, but may demonstrate intermittent displacement of the tendon.

Traumatic Luxation/Subluxation/ Ligament Injury

Ligament injuries of the tarsus usually result from severe trauma.

- A number of intertarsal injuries have been recognized as resulting from disruption of various ligament complexes between tarsal bones.
- Proximal intertarsal subluxation, proximal intertarsal luxation, and tarsometatarsal luxation are most common.

Signalment

- Any age or breed and either sex of dog or cat may be affected.

History

- Most animals are brought in for evaluation of a non-weight-bearing lameness.
- Some animals have an associated open wound over the tarsus.

Physical Examination

- Complete tarsocrural joint luxation is obvious; the animal is non-weight bearing and the paw deviates at an unnatural angle.
- Pain, swelling, and crepitus are present.

Diagnostic Imaging

- Standard craniocaudal and medial-to-lateral radiographs are often sufficient for complete evaluation (Figure 6.34).
- If instability is suspected but not confirmed, craniocaudal and varus–valgus stress films performed with the patient anesthetized are useful.

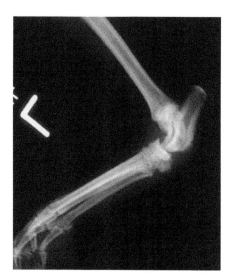

Figure 6.34 Radiographic indications of intertarsal subluxation.

IMPA, Poly-arthropathy

See Figure 6.35 and Chapter 5.

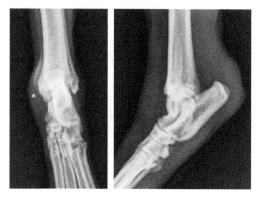

Figure 6.35 Radiographic indications of joint swelling (asterisk), associated with cytologic diagnosis of IMPA.

Digit Conditions

See Chapter 5.

Reference

Dewey, C.W., & da Costa, R.C. (2015). *Practical Guide to Canine and Feline Neurology*, 3rd ed. Chichester: Wiley-Blackwell.

Section 3

Case Discussion

7

Congenital/Developmental Conditions and Deformities

7.1   Congenital Elbow (Radial) Luxation

Case #1

Chief Complaint (CC): Unilateral thoracic limb lameness
Age: Young (onset at 3 months old, presented at 6 months old)
Size: Medium (21.4 kg at 6 months old), English Bulldog (Male (M))
Problem: Unilateral congenital elbow luxation (type I)

History

A 6-month-old English bulldog puppy presented for a right forelimb lameness and right elbow pain. He was adopted from a breeder.

- When he was 11 weeks old, he jumped from a chair and landed on his forelimbs. He started to limp on the right forelimb but a few days later, he seemed to have recovered from the injury and was not limping any more.
- Last week, while he was trying to jump on the owner, the owner had taken a step back and the puppy landed on his forelimbs on the ground. He started to limp on his right forelimb a few hours later and then he was in pain. He was taken to the vet the next morning, and the radiograph of the right elbow was taken. After luxation of the right radial head was identified, a closed reduction was attempted, which was not successful. Metacam injections were given. He is currently taking tramadol and something for the pain.

Physical Examination

- **Musculoskeletal**: Abnormal – non-weight-bearing lameness on right forelimb. Moderate swelling around the elbow and lateral luxation of radial head.
- **Nervous system**: Normal – normal cranial nerve function, proprioception.

Diagnostic Tests, Radiology/Computed Tomography (CT) Report

- Severe bilateral congenital elbow malformation with lateral radial luxation, incongruent humeroulnar joints, and mild osteoarthrosis. Right worse than left.
- Moderate soft tissue swelling, right thoracic limb.
- Probable healing type 1 Salter–Harris fracture, proximal right radius.

Diagnosis of Lameness in Dogs, First Edition. Edited by Kei Hayashi.
© 2023 John Wiley & Sons, Inc. Published 2023 by John Wiley & Sons, Inc.
Companion website: www.wiley.com/go/hayashi/lameness

- Bilateral, mild carpus valgus.
- Bilateral ulnar incomplete ossification, distal.

Conclusion

The recurrent right thoracic limb lameness is attributed to the cause of the soft tissue swelling and probable proximal radial physeal fracture, in addition to the underlying congenital elbow luxation. Soft tissue swelling in the right antebrachium may be attributed to the reported repetitive trauma, probable proximal radial fracture, and prior attempts to reduce the radial luxation; underlying cellulitis/infection is possible, but less likely given reported lack of fever.

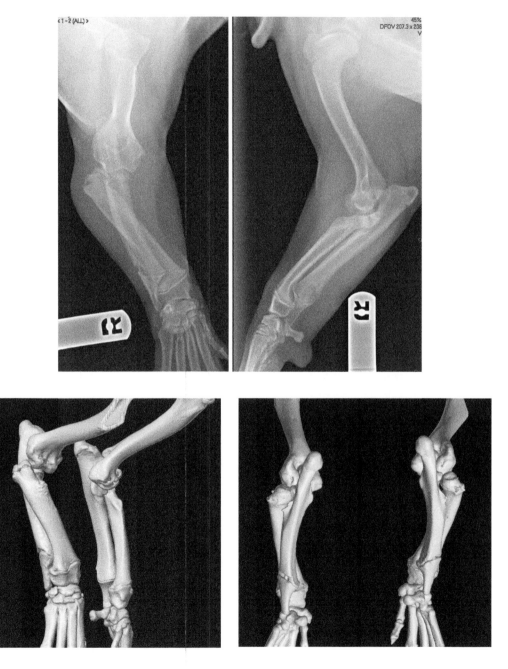

Case #2

CC: Thoracic limb lameness
Age: Young (5 months old)
Size: Medium (21.2 kg), Bulldog (M)
Problem: Angular limb deformity and elbow pain, elbow subluxation

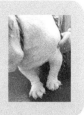

Video 7.1 Thoracic limb lameness (elbow subluxaion/angular limb deformity).

returned home from a trip. Additionally, his owners noticed a bowing appearance to the left limb.

- Radiographs revealed a suspected subluxation at the level of the humero-radial joint.

History

A 5-month-old male intact Bulldog presented for a two-week history of left thoracic limb lameness.

- His lameness was first noted two weeks prior to the presentation, after the owners

Physical Examination

- **Musculoskeletal**: Abnormal – left forelimb lameness with bowed appearance of left elbow. Painful on left elbow extension and flexion. Remainder of limbs palpated normally.

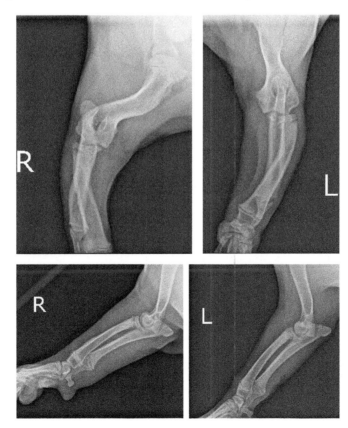

Case #3

CC: Thoracic limb deformity
Age: Young (onset at 3 months old, presented at 6 months old)
Size: Medium (10.7 kg at 6 months old), Bulldog/Shar Pei mix Female (F)
Problem: Unilateral congenital elbow luxation (type I) and angular limb deformity

Video 7.2 Mild gait abnormality (angular limb deformity/congenital elbow luxation).

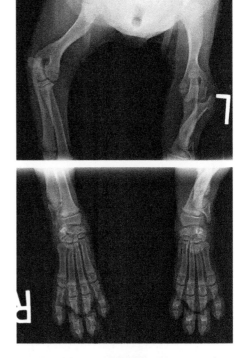

History

A 6-month-old female intact Bulldog/Shar Pei mix presented for a left thoracic limb deformity.

- At her purchase three months before (at about 3 months old), her owners noted that her left elbow "jutted out a little bit." Radiographs revealed several bony abnormalities in her left ulna and radius.
- A specialist examined the radiographs, and determined that her radial head is developing abnormally. They recommended a "wait and see" approach, and to use pain medications as necessary. They also recommended serial radiographs to assess changes with growth.
- At 3 months old, radiographs were taken.

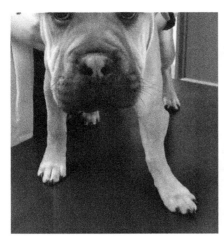

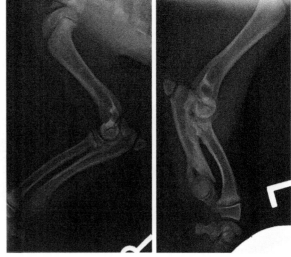

- At 5 months old, radiographs were repeated.

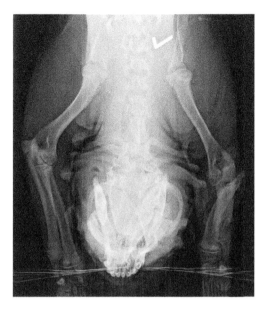

- She has had no pain or mobility limitations. She runs, jumps on and off the bed, uses the stairs, plays with the other 8-year-old dog in the home, and is generally a normal puppy.
- Her owners have noted that her elbow "sticks out more" and that her paw deviates, with her toes pointing laterally.

Physical Examination

- **Orthopedic exam**: Full range of motion, with no effusion, crepitus, or pain on flexion or extension in all four legs. No pain on long bone palpation in all four legs.
- **Left forelimb angular deformity**: Elbow laterally deviated, with radial head palpable on the lateral aspect of the elbow. Carpus medially deviated. Toes laterally deviated.

Video 7.3 Good elbow range of motion (congenital elbow luxation).

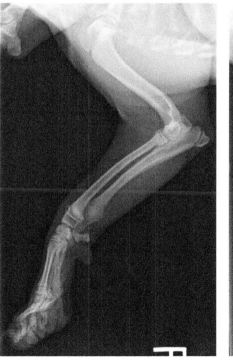

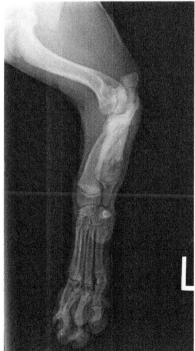

7.2 Congenital Elbow (Ulnar) Luxation

> **Case #4**
>
> **CC**: Bilateral thoracic limb deformity, nonambulatory
> **Age**: Young (onset: since birth, presented at 3 months old)
> **Size**: Medium (8.2 kg at 3 months old), Border Collie mix (M)
> **Problem**: Bilateral congenital elbow luxation (type II–III)

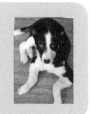

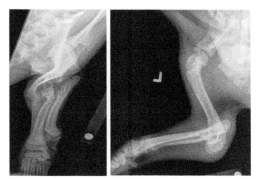

Video 7.4 Bilateral thoracic limb lameness/deformity (congenital elbow luxation).

History
A 3-month-old intact male Border Collie/ Cattle Dog mix presented for a severe bilateral congenital elbow deformity.

- He has had this deformity, in both elbows, since birth. Because of it, he cannot stand normally and has limited ambulatory ability. His current owners have had him for a week and a half.

Physical Examination
Bright, alert, and responsive, but not willing to walk with antebrachium on the ground.

- **Musculoskeletal**: Abnormal – bilateral forelimb deformities of the elbows.

Diagnostic Tests, Radiology/CT Report
Severe, bilaterally symmetric malformation and luxation, elbows.

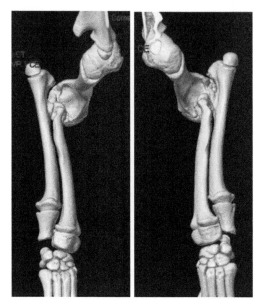

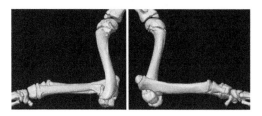

Case #5

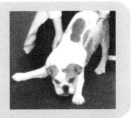

CC: Progressive bilateral thoracic limb lameness
Age: Young (onset at 3 months old, presented at 5 months old)
Size: Medium (11.7 kg at 5 months old), English Bulldog (F)
Problem: Bilateral congenital elbow luxation (type II–III)

Video 7.5 Bilateral thoracic limb lameness (congenital elbow luxation).

History

A 5-month-old intact female English Bulldog presented for evaluation of severe bilateral thoracic limb lameness.

- She was rescued from a breeder who believed she had "Swimmer Puppy Syndrome."
- Her primary veterinarian diagnosed her with a congenital bilateral elbow dysplasia, worse on the right. Initial radiographs revealed bilateral rotational abnormalities of the distal humerus and proximal radius/ulna with lateral ulnar luxation.
- She was prescribed carprofen 25 mg every 12 hours. Her foster mom notes that she is not overtly painful and plays with her housemates, but tires quickly and frequently bows her chest to the ground to rest.
- She is otherwise healthy with no episodes of coughing, sneezing, vomiting, or diarrhea.

Physical Examination

Bright, alert, and responsive, but not willing to walk with antebrachium on the ground.

- **Musculoskeletal**: Abnormal – elbows bilateral: lateral rotation of ulna/luxation, radius in place, rotational abnormality of distal humerus/proximal antebrachium, good joint stability, mildly decreased range of motion, no pain elicited on palpation, mild bilateral crepitus, no joint effusion, moderate muscle atrophy bilaterally in forelimbs. Bilateral forelimb weakness: bows chest to ground after taking a few steps. Remainder of musculature symmetric. No pain on long bone palpation.

Diagnostic Tests, Radiology/CT Report

- Bilateral elbow joint subluxation and malformation with mild osteoarthrosis.
- Questionable bilateral, bone fragments, supraglenoid tubercles.

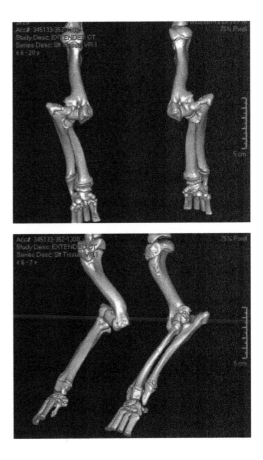

Case #6

CC: Progressive bilateral thoracic limb lameness
Age: Young (onset at 2–3 months old, presented at 4.5 months old)
Size: Medium (11.3 kg at 4.5 months old), Mixed (M)
Problem: Bilateral congenital elbow luxation (type II–III)

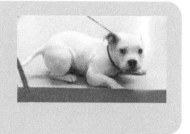

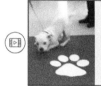

Video 7.6 Bilateral thoracic limb lameness (congenital elbow luxation).

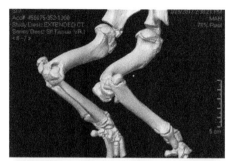

History

A 4.5-month-old, male intact, mixed-breed dog, presented for a bilateral congenital elbow abnormality.

- He was rescued from a shelter and now lives with a foster owner. He has been with the foster owner for three weeks. He has no history of surgery, is not on any medications nor has he received previous medications. He has not had any other medical issues.

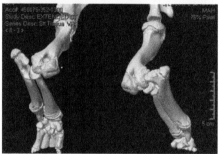

Physical Examination

Bright, alert, and responsive, but not willing to walk with antebrachium on the ground.

- **Musculoskeletal**: Abnormal – bilateral congenital luxation of elbows. Ambulates with forelimb splayed to sides and chest close to the ground in an "army crawl."

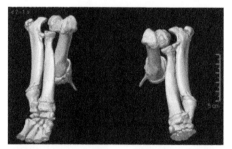

Diagnostic Tests, Radiology/CT Report

Severe bilateral elbow luxation with severe intracapsular swelling.

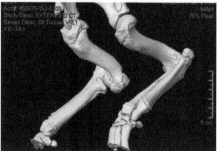

Case #7

CC: Bilateral thoracic limb deformity, nonambulatory
Age: Young (onset: since birth, presented at 7 months old)
Size: Medium (13.9 kg at 7 months old), Pitbull mix (M)
Problem: Bilateral congenital elbow luxation (type II–III)

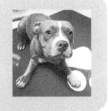

Video 7.7 Bilateral thoracic limb lameness/deformity (congenital elbow luxation).

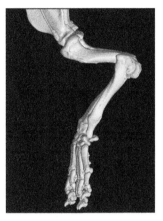

History

A 7-month-old intact male American Pitbull mix presented for previously diagnosed bilateral elbow luxation.

- He has had this deformity since birth. He is now being cared for by a rescue group.
- He is not on any medications and has no other known health issues.

Physical Examination

Bright, alert, and responsive, but not willing to walk with antebrachium on the ground.

- **Musculoskeletal**: Abnormal – bilaterally: forelimbs abducted. Walks slow. Luxated elbow – unknown bony involvement.

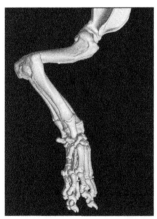

Diagnostic Tests, Radiology/CT Report

- Severe, bilateral elbow dysplasia with bilateral lateral dislocation (luxation) of the proximal aspect of the ulna.
- Retained cartilaginous core, left distal ulnar physis.

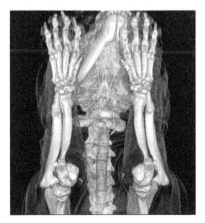

7.3 Angular Limb Deformity/Elbow Subluxation

Case #8

CC: Thoracic limb lameness, deformity, bilateral (worse on the right)
Age: Young (onset at 3 months old, presented at 1 year old)
Size: Medium (22 kg at 1 year), Basset Hound (chondrodystrophic breed) Neutered Male (NM)
Problem: Angular limb deformity and elbow subluxation/dysplasia (medial coronoid disease)

History

A 1-year-old male castrated Basset Hound presented for a deformity in his right front leg that has progressively gotten worse for around 7 months, since he was 3 months old.

- His right front paw twists and rotates while he walks, causing him to fall down occasionally.
- Radiographs (6 weeks prior) revealed abnormalities in both front limbs, with the left limb being mild.

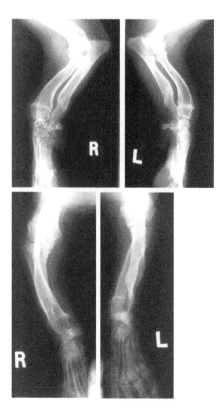

Physical Examination

- **Musculoskeletal**: Abnormal – internal rotation of right front carpus with snapping motion that disrupted his balance at a faster pace; Significant head bobbing movement; Pain with palpation and maximal extension of his right and left elbows; Grade 1 lateral patellar luxation noted on his right hind limb.

Diagnostic Tests, Radiology/CT Report

- Moderate incongruity with moderate to severe radial subluxation and moderate osteoarthrosis, left elbow.
- Mild incongruity right humeroulnar.
- Mild to moderate bilateral carpal vagus.
- Mild bilateral otitis externa.

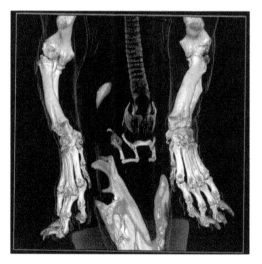

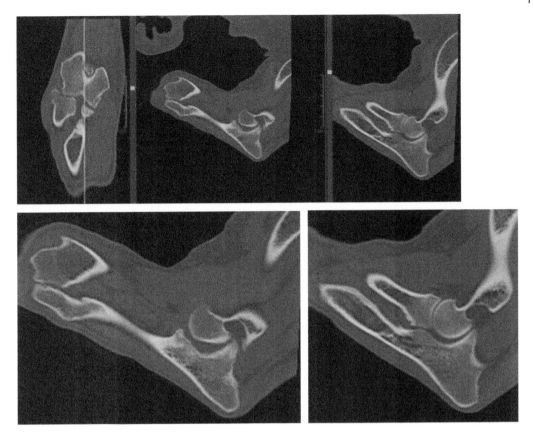

CT: Left elbow subluxation, distal ulnar physeal closure.

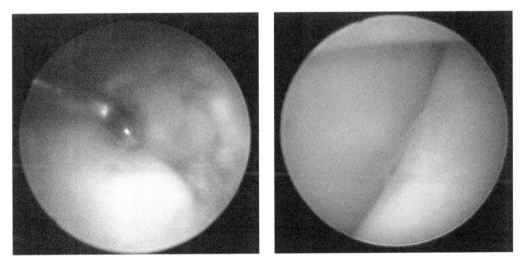

Arthroscopy: Damaged medial coronoid process (left) and anconeal process (right).

Case #9

CC: Thoracic limb deformity and lameness
Age: Young (7 months old)
Size: Small (2.64 kg at 7 months old), Chihuahua (NM)
Problem: Premature closure of distal ulnar physis, angular limb deformity, elbow subluxation

Video 7.8 Thoracic limb lameness (angular limb deformity).

History

A 7-month-old male intact long-haired Chihuahua presented for left front-limb lameness.

- Two months ago (at 5 months old), he began holding up his left front limb while running, and his owner noticed that the left front seemed bowed outward slightly.
- Radiographs showed closed physis on the left distal ulna and open physis on the right limb. He was nonpainful on palpation of the leg.

- The limping has not changed since then. He occasionally stands on the limb, but lifts the limb when running.

Physical Examination
- **Musculoskeletal**: Abnormal – stands x4 but when running limps on the left front or holds it in the air. Nonpainful on palpation. Open fontanel on head. Neuro exam within normal limits (WNL).

Diagnostic Tests, Radiology/CT Report
- Asynchronous growth of the left radius and ulna with severe elbow subluxation and moderate carpal valgus.
- Questionable bilateral metaphyseal abnormality.

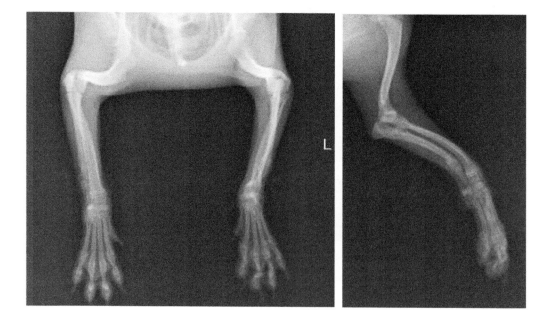

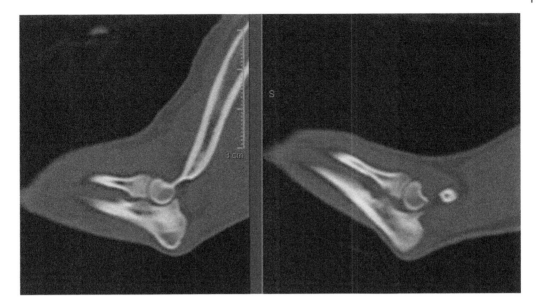

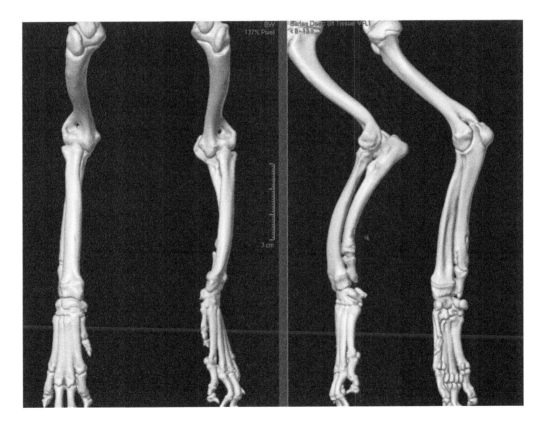

Case #10

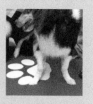

CC: Thoracic limb deformity, bilateral
Age: Young (7 months old)
Size: Medium (20.0 kg at 7 months old), Collie (M)
Problem: Bilateral angular limb deformity, elbow dysplasia (osteochondritis dissecans, medial coronoid disease)

History

A 7-month-old intact male Collie, presented for evaluation of bilateral forelimb angular limb deformity.

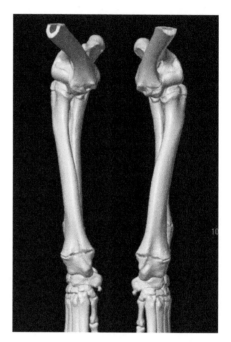

- Owners first noticed his forelimbs were not straight when he was adopted five months before (at 2 months old). At that time, the angulation was mild and after assessment by the primary care veterinarian, it was determined that the angulation was not worrisome.
- He walks and runs comfortably at home, but his forelimbs seems to be worsening.

Physical Examination

- **Musculoskeletal**: Abnormal – bilateral forelimb angular limb abnormalities, effusion of the right elbow, painful elbows on palpation, swelling both elbows, no elbow luxation identified at this time.

Diagnostic Tests, Radiology/CT Report

- Bilateral angular thoracic limb deformity.
- Bilateral elbow dysplasia (humeral trochlea osteochondritis dissecans [OCD], moderate elbow joint incongruence, and mild osteoarthritis).
- Mild left flexor enthesopathy.

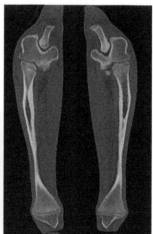

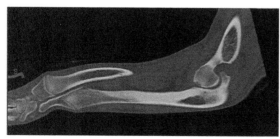

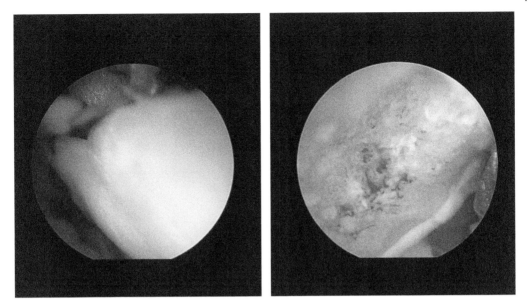

Arthroscopy: OCD (left) and OCD bed after debridement (right).

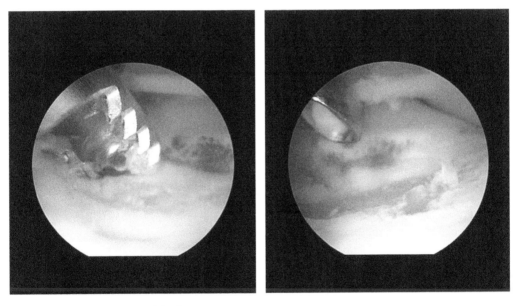

Medial coronoid process after debridement.

Case #11

CC: Thoracic limb lameness, deformity, bilateral (worse on the right)
Age: Young (onset at 4 months old, presented at 1 year old)
Size: Medium (26.5 kg at 1 year), mixed (NM)
Problem: Angular limb deformity and elbow subluxation (incongruity)

Video 7.9 Thoracic limb lameness (angular limb deformity).

History

A 1-year-old male castrated mixed-breed dog, presented for evaluation of a right forelimb lameness and angular limb deformity.

- His owners adopted him 6 months before (at about 4 months old) and noticed mild angulation of his right forelimb. The limb angulation continued to worsen.
- He is able to run around and jump off things without significant clinical signs. He gets glucosamine supplements twice a day.

Physical Examination

- **Musculoskeletal**: Abnormal – right forelimb carpal valgus and elbow varus due to radial lateral angulation, decreased right carpal flexion and flexion of right elbow. Left mild carpal valgus, normal range of movement, pelvic limbs palpated normally.

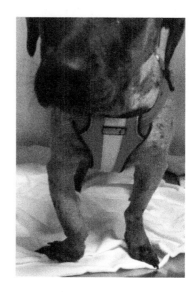

Diagnostic Tests, Radiology/CT Report

The patient has bilateral asynchronous growth of the radius and ulna with severe external rotation/valgus deformity of the manus (right>left), severe elbow incongruency with moderate to severe osteoarthrosis, intraarticular osteochondral fragments (right), bilateral medial coronoid disease, mild right flexor enthesopathy, and mild right antebrachiocarpal degenerative joint disease. A cause for the asynchronous growth is not determined during this evaluation and the differential diagnosis includes trauma and genetic causes.

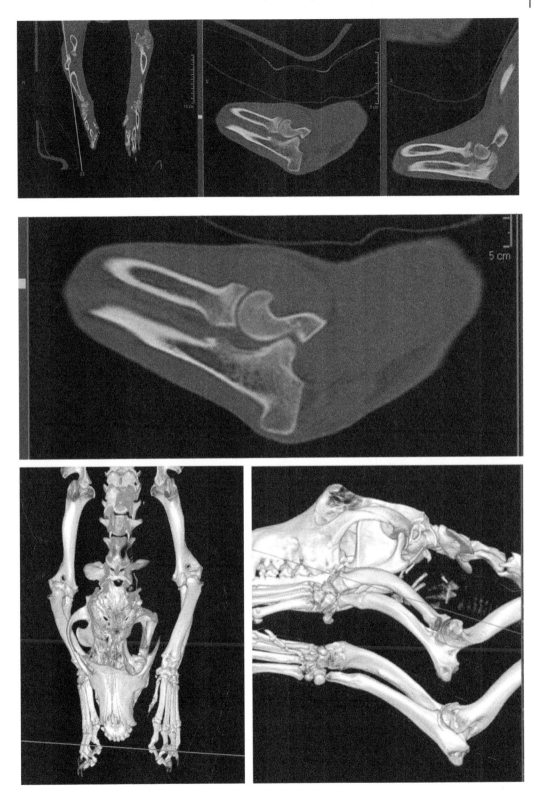

Case #12

CC: Thoracic limb deformity and lameness
Age: Young (5 months old)
Size: Large (20.8 kg at 5 months old), German Shepherd (F)
Problem: Unilateral angular limb deformity, physeal fracture, premature closure of distal ulnar physis, asymmetric premature closure of distal radial physis

Video 7.10 Thoracic limb deformity/lameness (angular limb deformity).

History

A 5-month-old female intact German Shepherd dog, presented for evaluation of a left forelimb angular limb deformity.

- Three months ago (at 2 months old), she injured her left second metacarpal bone after jumping off the bed. The injury was splinted and healed over a three-week period.

- One month ago (at 4 months old), two weeks after the splint removal, the owners noted an angular deviation of her left forelimb. The limb was radiographed and a suspected type V Salter–Harris fracture of the distal ulnar physis was suspected.

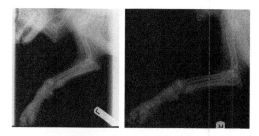

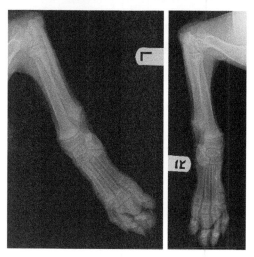

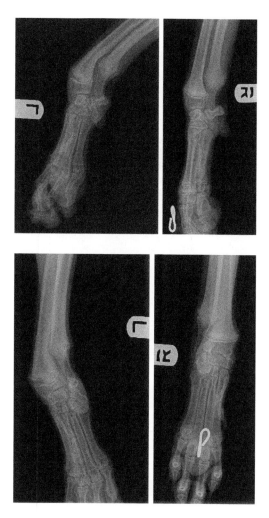

- The patient was then referred to an orthopedic surgeon. In the past, she has been prescribed carprofen, but did not improve. Otherwise, she is healthy, up to date on vaccinations, and eats Blue Buffalo puppy food.

Physical Examination

- **Musculoskeletal**: Abnormal – left forelimb muscle atrophy, left forelimb lameness, left carpal valgus, crepitus at left elbow, CN WNL, spinal reflexes WNL, CP x 4 WNL.

Diagnostic Tests, Radiology/CT Report

- Asynchronous growth of the left radius and ulna due to premature closure of the distal ulnar physis.
- Mild elbow incongruence and carpal valgus, left.
- Mild to moderate muscle atrophy, left thoracic limb.
- Chronic healed fractures, second and third metacarpal bones, left.

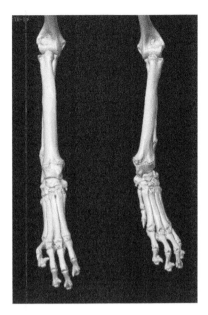

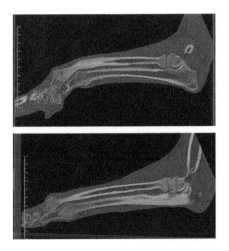

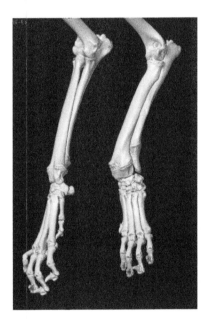

7.4 Carpal Laxity Syndrome

> ### Case #13
>
> **CC**: Thoracic limb lameness, bilateral deformity
> **Age**: Young (onset at 2 months old, presented at 3 months old)
> **Size**: Medium (7.2 kg at 3 months), English Bulldog (M)
> **Problem**: Carpal laxity

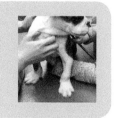

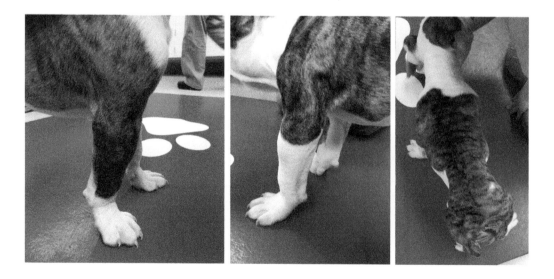

Video 7.11 Dropped carpus (carpal laxity).

History

A 3-month-old male intact English Bulldog presenting for right front-limb lameness starting about 3–4 weeks ago and not improving.

- He appears to walk on his "elbows," which worsens when playing and active. Owner has restricted activity to kennel, which seems to help. He does not appear painful but will lay down when his front-leg lameness worsens. He has no obvious problems with his back legs, but walks abnormally.

- He is from a litter of eight pups from the owner's female dog. One of the pups in the litter passed.
- He was born with a cleft lip, which has not caused any problems and does not extend into the palate. The owner plans on addressing the cleft lip at a later date. No other pups have any problems identified.
- Breathes well at home, no snoring/snorting/coughing.
- Very active at home and wants to play constantly. No medications/supplements.

Physical Examination

Ambulatory x4 with carpal laxity/hyperextension (R>L). Hind-limb varus. Good, symmetric musculature. No pain on long bone palpation. No joint effusion, pain, or crepitus appreciated. Full range of motion x4.

Case #14

CC: Unilateral thoracic limb lameness and deformity
Age: Young (onset at 2 months old, presented at 3 months old)
Size: Large, Labradoodle (M)
Problem: Carpal laxity

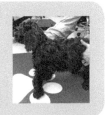

 Video 7.12 Carpal "buckling" (carpal laxity/flexural deformtiy).

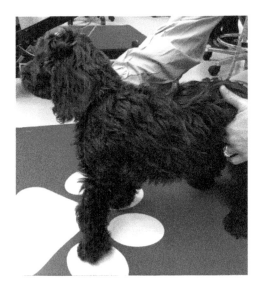

History

An 11 week-old male intact Labradoodle, presented for progressive lameness and bow-legged bilateral front legs. The owner noticed that the right front leg was bow-legged 3–4 weeks ago. The patient was taken to a veterinarian for radiographs and was thought to have a fracture. The leg was splinted and wrapped for 5 days. The wrap was removed 5 days later with no follow-up radiographs, but no improvement in the leg was noted. The left forelimb also became bowed two weekends ago. He is otherwise a happy and healthy puppy and does not appear to be in any pain.

- He is currently being housed by himself in a kennel or crate and his activity has been restricted to prevent further injury.
- None of the other dogs in his litter has developed deformities in its limbs, although two of them seem to shake their front limbs frequently.

Physical Examination

- **Musculoskeletal**: Abnormal – bow-legged appearance of the forelimbs bilaterally when standing.
- Carpal flexion while standing, resulting in a broken-over appearance bilaterally in the carpi (left worse than right), with extension of the digits and normal weight bearing.
- No pain, effusion, or crepitus on palpation of the carpi. No pain, effusion, or crepitus noted in any additional joints. No long bone pain on palpation.

7.5   Genu Recurvatum (Congenital Stifle Hyperextension)

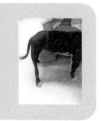

Case #15

CC: Unilateral pelvic limb lameness
Age: Young (onset unknown, presented at 4 months old)
Size: Medium (7.6 kg at 4 months), Pitbull mix (spayed female (SF))
Problem: Stifle hyperextension

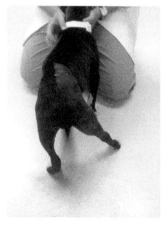

Video 7.13 Pelvic limb lameness (stifle hyperextensio).

History

An approximately 4-month-old female spayed mixed-breed dog for surgical correction of left pelvic limb genu recurvatum. History prior to her rescue is limited.

- Prior to her rescue, she has constantly held her left hind limb in extension with her femur externally rotated.
- She is unable to flex her stifle, even to a normal standing position.

- She has been eating well and seems otherwise healthy, but has no functional use of her left hind limb.

Physical Examination

- **Musculoskeletal**: Abnormal – right hind limb held in extension, externally rotated with quadriceps contracture, medial luxation of the patella (grade 4), decreased mobility of tarsal joint.
- **Nervous system**: Normal – no proprioceptive deficits; full exam not performed.

Diagnostic Tests, Radiology/CT Report

Moderate external rotation and hyperextension of the limb with moderate medial patellar luxation, right pelvic limb.

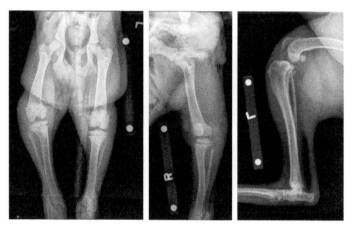

Case #16

CC: Unilateral pelvic limb lameness
Age: Young (onset since birth, presented at 2.5 months old)
Size: Large (6.2 kg at 2.5 months), German Shepherd (F)
Problem: Stifle hyperextension, Hip subluxation

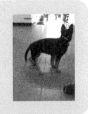

Video 7.14 Pelvic limb lameness (stifle hyperextensio).

History

German Shepherd dog presented for right hind-limb dysfunction.

- Since her birth, she has had hyperextension of her stifle and tarsal joints.
- Radiographs reveal subluxation of her right hip joint.
- Her activity level has been normal, she shows no evidence of pain while ambulating, and she readily plays with the other dog in her home.
- She is otherwise healthy and has begun her puppy vaccination series.

Physical Examination

- **Musculoskeletal**: Abnormal – severe hyperextension of right stifle and right tarsus, pain elicited upon stifle flexion.
- **Nervous system**: Not evaluated fully – appropriate mentation, delayed correction on right hindlimb likely due to muscle contracture.

Diagnostic Tests, Radiology/CT Report

Severe right genu recurvatum with secondary right-hip subluxation.

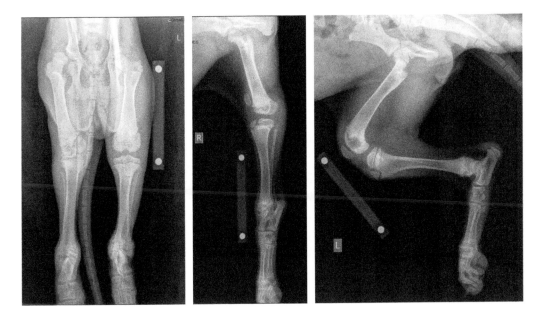

7.6 Tibial Deformity (Pes Varus)

> **Case #17**
>
> **CC**: Unilateral pelvic limb lameness
> **Age**: Young (onset since birth, presented at 10 months old)
> **Size**: Small (6.0 kg at 15 months), Miniature Dachshund (NM)
> **Problem**: Unilateral tibial deformity

History
Since his birth, he has had a bowed-leg appearance on his right hind leg. No obvious lameness.

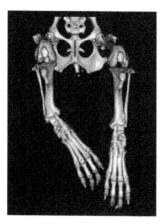

Physical Examination
- **Musculoskeletal**: Normal range of motion. No pain. Varus at tarsal joint.
- **Nervous system**: Normal.

Diagnostic Tests, Radiology/CT Report
Pes varus, tibia vara, right.

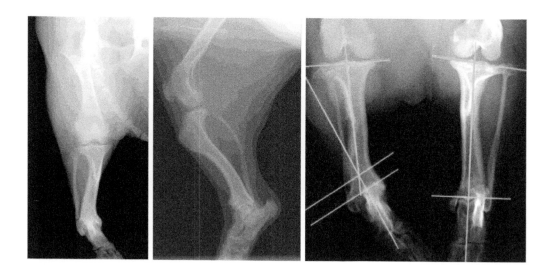

7.7 Hypertrophic Osteodystrophy

Case #18

CC: Leg swellings and decreased appetite
Age: Young (onset at 5 months old, presented at 7 months old)
Size: Giant (34.5 kg at 7 months), Great Dane (F)
Problem: Hypertrophic osteodystrophy (all four limbs)

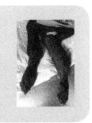

History

A 7-month-old female intact Great Dane presented for a two-month history of leg swellings and decreased appetite.

- About 3 months ago, she was noted to have difficulty walking. Dog food she was on as a puppy – commercial diet. Vaccines as a puppy – needed third series.
- She was taken to an emergency care veterinarian for evaluation. It was noted at the time that her joints were sensitive to palpation and warm to the touch. No radiographs were taken during this episode and she was subsequently diagnosed with panosteitis.
- She was given intravenous fluid therapy, 2.25 mL famotidine subcutaneously, 0.6 mL meloxicam subcutaneously, and sent home on 75 mg meloxicam 1/2 tab orally once daily for six days.
- One week later, she returned to the emergency room for reluctance to walk. Radiographs were offered, but declined at this time, and she was treated again with meloxicam and famotidine for six days.
- Two weeks later, radiographs of her affected limbs were taken and she was diagnosed with hypertrophic osteodystrophy. She was started on Deramaxx 75 mg 1/2 tab once a day for 14 days, and was ordered to have strict cage rest and to be fed a giant-breed puppy food. Deramaxx didn't seem to improve her. She was given CBD oil, no walks. Lays around in her house.
- Today, she returns for being extremely painful, anorexic, and lethargic. She is still receiving Deramaxx 1 mg/kg orally once a day.

Physical Examination

- **Musculoskeletal**: Full orthopedic examination limited due to patient painful upon touching swellings. Patient ambulatory on presentation, but hesitant to walk, gait abnormal due to large swellings, and possible deformities associated with the swellings. Once sedated, more extensive orthopedic examination was performed. Patient was noted to have very large, firm swellings primarily at the distal metaphyseal region of L/R radius/ulna and L/R tibia. Medial aspect of the distal metaphyseal region of the left femur was also noted to be swollen.
- **Nervous system**: Full neuro exam not performed due to patient's pain. No overt neuropathies noted on examination.

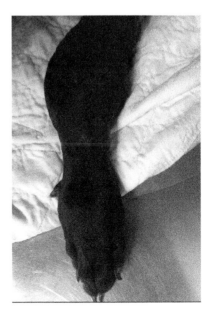

Diagnostic Tests, Radiology/CT Report

Moderate to severe, generalized polyostotic osteopathy.

- In the left femur and left tibia, the proximal and distal metaphyses have moderate to severe, both smoothly and irregularly margined, periosteal proliferation and sclerosis. The periosteal proliferation extends to, but does not overtly cross, the physes.

- The soft tissues surrounding the proximal and distal diaphyses of the left tibia and femur are moderately to severely, locally extensively, thick.

- Impression: Lameness and radiographic findings are attributed to hypertrophic osteodystrophy.

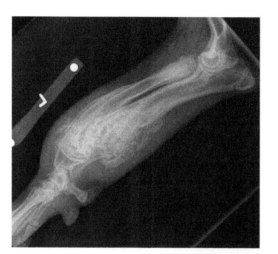

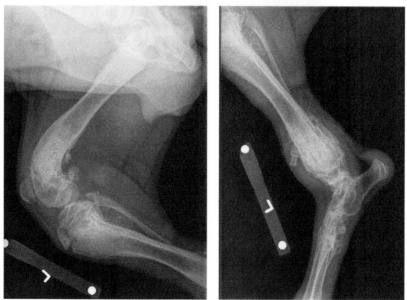

The videos are available for this chapter on www.wiley.com/go/hayashi/lameness.

8

Thoracic Limb Lameness in Young Dogs

8.1 Elbow Dysplasia (Medial Coronoid Disease)

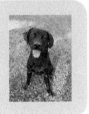

Case #1

Chief Complaint (CC): Left thoracic limb lameness
Age: Young (10 months old)
Size: Large (29.5 kg), Labrador Retriever (M)
Problem: Elbow dysplasia (medial coronoid disease/fissure)

Video 8.1 Thoracic limb lameness (elbow dysplasia).

History

A 10-month-old male Labrador presented for evaluation for left thoracic limb lameness.

- Last week, he slipped on the kitchen floor and went acutely lame in his front left limb. He was rested over the weekend to see if it would resolve.

Physical Examination

- **Musculoskeletal**: Abnormal – gait: wide thoracic gait, grade 2/5 lame in the left thoracic limb, ambulatory x4; no overt ataxia. Left thoracic limb: small amount of effusion felt in the left elbow, normal range of movement at each joint, small amount of pain upon deep elbow palpation, no long bone pain. Right thoracic limb: normal. Pelvic limbs: normal.
- **Nervous system**: Normal – appropriate mentation; normal cranial nerves (pupillary light reflex [PLR], menace, palpebral); normal conscious proprioception; full neuro exam not performed, no nystagmus or strabismus noted; no ataxia.

Diagnostic Tests, Radiology/Computed Tomography (CT) Report

Mild medial coronoid disease.

Diagnosis of Lameness in Dogs, First Edition. Edited by Kei Hayashi.
© 2023 John Wiley & Sons, Inc. Published 2023 by John Wiley & Sons, Inc.
Companion website: www.wiley.com/go/hayashi/lameness

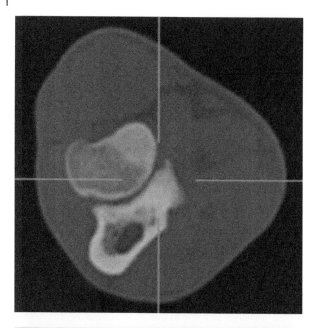

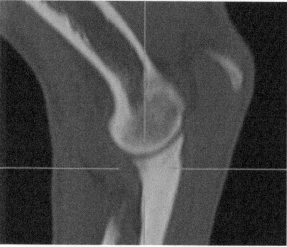

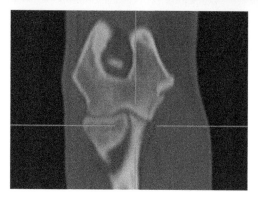

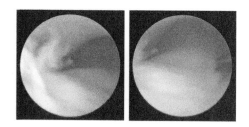

Arthroscopy: mild medial coronoid disease (chondromalacia and superficial fissure).

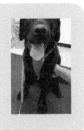

Case #2

CC: Bilateral thoracic limb lameness (worse on the right)
Age: Young (onset at 11 months old, presented at 12 months old)
Size: Large (36.1 kg), Labrador Retriever (NM)
Problem: Elbow dysplasia (medial coronoid disease/fragmented coronoid process)

Video 8.2 Thoracic limb lameness (elbow dysplasia) [Slow Motion].

History

A 1-year-old, male neutered English Labrador presented for evaluation for thoracic limb lameness.

- He has a one-month history of bilateral thoracic limb lameness, reported as worse on the right limb.
- He had been previously evaluated by two veterinarians who diagnosed him with bilateral elbow dysplasia and recommended surgery. He was put on 300 mg gabapentin until this visit.
- He was neutered at 8 months.
- He receives Dasuquin once a day with his morning meal. He had diarrhea shortly after starting gabapentin, but his veterinarian prescribed metronidazole due to suspected dietary indiscretion and this has since resolved.

Physical Examination

- **Musculoskeletal**: Abnormal – ambulatory x4; elbow effusion bilaterally but worse on the right; pain elicited on elbow extension and flexion bilaterally; mild cranial drawer bilaterally; no tibial thrust bilaterally; shifting forelimb lameness at a walk.

Diagnostic Tests, Radiology/CT Report

- Moderate to severe medial coronoid disease (with fragmentation), moderate elbow osteoarthrosis, and mild flexor enthesopathy, both elbows.
- The results of this evaluation are positive for elbow dysplasia, to which bilateral forelimb lameness is attributed.

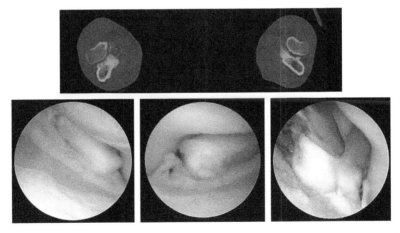

Arthroscopy: medial coronoid disease (fragmented coronoid process, full-thickness cartilage defect, and "kissing lesion" in humeral condyle).

Case #3

CC: Bilateral thoracic limb lameness
Age: Young (onset at 6 months old, presented at 1 year and 8 months old)
Size: Large (33.7 kg), Bernese Mountain Dog (SF)
Problem: Elbow dysplasia (medial coronoid disease/fragmented coronoid process)

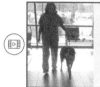

Video 8.3 Thoracic limb lameness (elbow dysplasia).

History

A 20-month-old, female spayed Bernese Mountain Dog presented for forelimb lameness and treatment of suspected elbow dysplasia.

- When she was about 6 months old, her owner began to notice her limping on her right front leg after playing in the yard or going on walks. At times she hops and is completely non-weight bearing on the right front limb.
- Her primary vet attributed this to growing too fast and recommended reducing protein in her diet.
- The lameness has not improved, and two weeks ago she had radiographs performed by her primary vet and a specialist. She was also prescribed Cosequin and 75 mg Deramaxx to be given once daily as needed. She has received the Cosequin daily for the past two weeks, and has only received Deramaxx after intense exercise and anticipated pain. The last dose of Deramaxx was given about 1 week ago.
- She is a picky eater, but has good energy levels. She is otherwise healthy according to her owner and is on no other medications.

Physical Examination

- **Musculoskeletal**: Bilateral forelimb lameness. Bilateral elbow effusion, worse on the right. Crepitus on flexion and extension of both elbows. Pain on palpation of medial coronoid process bilaterally. Hind limbs normal.

Diagnostic Tests, Radiology/CT Report

- Severe bilateral elbow arthropathy.
- The results of this evaluation are positive for elbow dysplasia and severe bilateral elbow osteoarthrosis, to which bilateral thoracic limb lameness is attributed.

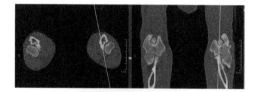

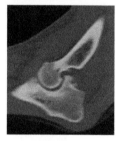

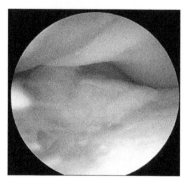

Arthroscopy: medial coronoid disease (fragmented coronoid process, full-thickness cartilage defect, and "kissing lesion" in humeral condyle).

Case #4

CC: Right thoracic limb lameness
Age: Young (onset at 7 months old, presented at 11 months old)
Size: Large (38.3 kg at 11 months old), Labrador Retriever (NM)
Problem: Bilateral elbow dysplasia (medial coronoid disease/fragmented coronoid process), hip dysplasia

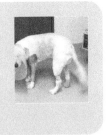

History

An 11-month-old male castrated Labrador Retriever presented for a history of lameness and suspected elbow dysplasia.

- Ever since he was a puppy, when the owners acquired him from a breeder at 8 weeks old, they noticed that he bunny hops in the back and has trouble with stairs.
- He sometimes has trouble getting up off the floor and when he lays down, his carpi appear contracted.
- When he was 7 months old, he was being boarded at a kennel and the staff noticed that he was quite lame in the front, and he was presented to a veterinarian for workup.
- Radiographs showed questionable signs of elbow dysplasia and physical exam revealed pain on hyperextension of the elbows. Radiographs of the pelvis were normal at that time.
- He goes to work with his owner daily. He also lives with one other dog, two cats, and a turtle.

Physical Examination

- **Musculoskeletal**: Mild (2/6) lameness right hind, moderate (3/6) lameness right fore. Ambulatory x4. Pain on extension of both elbows. Questionable cranial drawer and tibial thrust positive left stifle. Decreased range of movement/pain on right hip.

Diagnostic Tests, Radiology/CT Report

- Moderate to severe medial coronoid disease with fragmentation and moderate osteoarthrosis, left ulna.
- Moderate medial coronoid disease with fragmentation and moderate osteoarthrosis, right ulna.
- Persistent lameness is attributed to the listed abnormalities. The results of this evaluation are positive for elbow dysplasia.

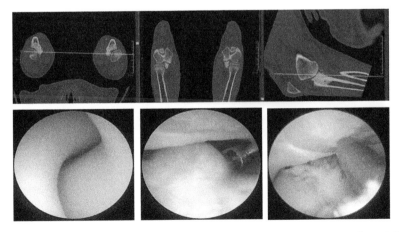

Arthroscopy: Medial coronoid disease (fragmented coronoid process, full-thickness cartilage defect, and "kissing lesion" in humeral condyle).

8.2 Shoulder Osteochondrosis Dissecans

Case #5

CC: Right thoracic limb lameness
Age: Young (6 months old)
Size: Medium (13.2 kg at 6 months old), Border Collie (F)
Problem: Shoulder osteochondrosis dissecans (OCD), unilateral

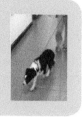

Video 8.4 Thoracic limb lameness (shoulder OCD).

Diagnostic Tests, Radiology/CT Report
Not available.

History

A 6-month-old intact female Border Collie presented for evaluation of her right forelimb lameness.

- Four weeks ago, she became lame on her right forelimb and was taken to her primary veterinarian for further evaluation after a week of no improvement.
- Shoulder radiographs revealed an OCD lesion of her right proximal humerus. She is otherwise healthy and has no past medical conditions.

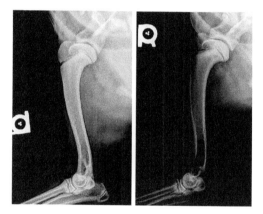

Physical Examination

- **Musculoskeletal**: Mild lameness on right thoracic limb, mild pain on flexion and extension of right shoulder. Normal muscle tone and symmetry bilaterally.

Arthroscopy: Shoulder OCD flap (left) and bed (right).

Case #6

CC: Right thoracic limb lameness
Age: Young (onset before 5 months old, presented at 12 months old)
Size: Giant (46.4 kg at 12 months old), St. Bernard (SF)
Problem: Shoulder osteochondrosis dissecans (OCD, bilateral, worse on the right)

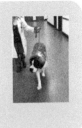

Video 8.5 Thoracic limb lameness (shoulder OCD).

History

A 1-year-old, female spayed St. Bernard dog, for evaluation of right forelimb lameness.

- She becomes lame on her leg any time she plays or is active for as long as her owners have had her (since she was a very young puppy).
- She has been on glucosamine chondroitin for several months and her owners have not seen any improvement in her lameness.
- She lives on a farm with other animals, but no other animals live in the house with her.

- She is on 1 tablet of glucosamine chondroitin and no other medications.

Physical Examination

- **Musculoskeletal**: Abnormal – marked right forelimb lameness at walk. Pain elicited on extension and flexion of right shoulder joint. Muscle atrophy of shoulder muscles on right side. In hind limbs, normal bilaterally symmetric musculature. No evidence of long bone pain, joint effusion, or instability. No evidence of cervical, thoracic, or lumbosacral discomfort.

Diagnostic Tests, Radiology/CT Report

- Bilateral osteochondritis dissecans.
- Mild, right shoulder osteoarthrosis.
- The results of this examination confirm the presence of bilateral shoulder OCD.

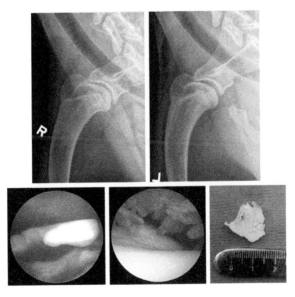

Arthroscopy: Shoulder OCD flap/bed (left), synovitis (middle), and removed flap (right).

8.3 Physeal Fractures, Avulsion Fractures

Case #7

CC: Acute right thoracic limb lameness
Age: Young (7 months old)
Size: Small (3.4 kg at 7 months old), Yorkshire Terrier (SF)
Problem: Salter–Harris type 1 distal radius fracture

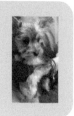

History

A 7-month-old female spayed Yorkshire Terrier jumped off the owners' bed and ran into the edge of the open door.

- She was non-weight bearing on her right front limb.
- Owners were given meloxicam (0.5 mg/mL, 1 mL q24) and Tramadol (1/4 of 50 mg tablet q8). The owners believe the medications have helped with her pain. She has had two episodes of diarrhea since being started on the medications.

- She has been eating, drinking, and urinating normally, with no coughing episodes.

Physical Examination

- **Musculoskeletal**: Not evaluated – right forelimb is splinted; non-weight bearing.

Diagnostic Tests, Radiology/CT Report

- Acute, traumatic Salter–Harris fracture type 1, distal right radius and ulna.

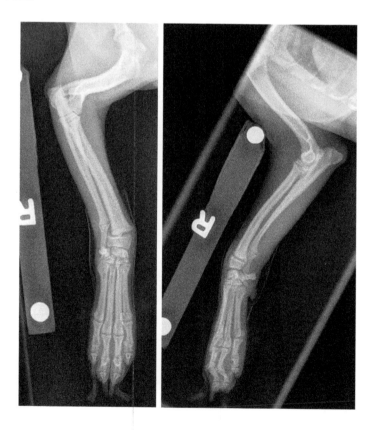

Case #8

CC: Chronic right thoracic limb lameness
Age: Young (6 months old)
Size: Medium (13.1 kg at 6 months old), Australian Shepherd (F)
Problem: Supraglenoid tubercle avulsion fracture

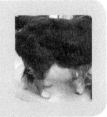

History

A 6-month-old intact female Australian Shepherd presented for evaluation of right front-limb lameness.

- About one month ago, she slipped while trying to jump over an obstacle on a hike, falling with her right front limb caudally and her left front limb cranially. She was immediately non-weight bearing lame afterward, and was presented to her primary veterinarian the following day.
- She was prescribed two different courses of carprofen, which seemed to help with the lameness, and also received 10 cold laser therapy treatments, which did not seem to help with the lameness.
- She was kenneled for one week while her owner was out of town, and seemed better after this week of rest. She has especially improved in the past two weeks.
- She is not exhibiting any signs of systemic illness and is not currently receiving pain medication (last dose one month ago), or any other medications or supplements.
- She has not gone on any additional hikes with her owner.

Physical Examination

- **Musculoskeletal**: Standing examination right front limb: mild antebrachial muscle atrophy, pain upon abduction of shoulder joint.

Diagnostic Tests, Radiology/CT Report

- Articular avulsion fracture, right supraglenoid tubercle.

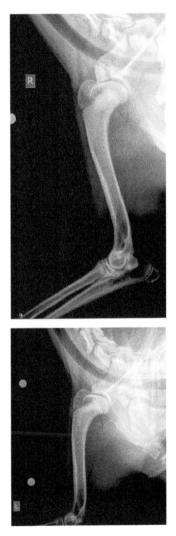

The videos are available for this chapter on www.wiley.com/go/hayashi/lameness.

9

Thoracic Limb Lameness in Mature Dogs

9.1 Elbow Osteoarthritis

Case #1

Chief Complaint (CC): Chronic right thoracic limb lameness
Age: Mature (5 years old)
Size: Medium (25.8 kg), Pitbull Terrier (SF)
Problem: Chronic elbow osteoarthritis (OA) secondary to elbow dysplasia (medial coronoid disease/fragmented coronoid process)

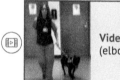

Video 9.1 Thoracic limb lameness (elbow OA).

History

An almost 5-year-old female spayed Staffordshire Terrier presented for evaluation of a forelimb lameness.

- The patient was adopted at 2.5 years old. She was noted to be healthy at that time with no immediate concerns.
- Four months ago, it was appreciated that she was lame in her forelimbs, most notably the right. At this time she was still running around and playing with a normal energy level and going on two 20-minute walks daily.

- She was seen by her primary care veterinarian where radiographs of her elbows were taken (radiographs not available for review). At that time she was started on Galliprant and tramadol. Since starting the medications, her lameness has dramatically improved; however, her leash walk time has been reduced.
- No systemic health concerns appreciated by owner.

Physical Examination
- **Orthopedic examination**
  - Gait analysis:
    - Grade 3–4/5 right forelimb lameness, minimal lameness on left forelimb.
    - Limb length discrepancy, with hindlimbs subjectively taller than forelimbs, creating sway back.

Diagnosis of Lameness in Dogs, First Edition. Edited by Kei Hayashi.
© 2023 John Wiley & Sons, Inc. Published 2023 by John Wiley & Sons, Inc.
Companion website: www.wiley.com/go/hayashi/lameness

- ○ Right hip hike noted at a trot with abaxial placement of right hindlimb during gait cycling.
- ○ Hind limbs had minimal flexion throughout the gait cycle (R>L).

- Standing exam
  - ○ Right forelimb abduction with external rotation and carpal valgus.
  - ○ Weight shifting to left limbs, offloading right forelimb and hindlimb.
  - ○ Right shoulder muscle spasm on direct palpation and multiple muscle knots on the cranial boarder of the scapula.
  - ○ Forelimb muscle atrophy, R>L – especially of triceps musculature.
  - ○ Bilateral elbow thickening with remodeling and mild effusion bilaterally, R>L.
  - ○ Hypertrophy of flexor tendons on left forelimb.

- ○ Thoraco-lumbar kyphosis with paralumbar muscle spasms on direct palpation.
- ○ Bilateral hindlimb atrophy, R>L.
- ○ Keeping right hindlimb extended ("straight").

- Recumbent exam
  - ○ Decreased elbow flexion>extension with crepitus and discomfort on end range of movement, R>L.
  - ○ Resistant to hip abduction and end extension with mild discomfort, R>L.
- **Neurologic exam**: No abnormal findings.

Diagnostic Tests, Radiology/Computed Tomography (CT) Report
- **Bilateral, severe elbow dysplasia** (united anconeal processes, medial coronoid disease with right-sided fragmentation) with severe, chronic degenerative joint disease and intracapsular swelling (R>L).

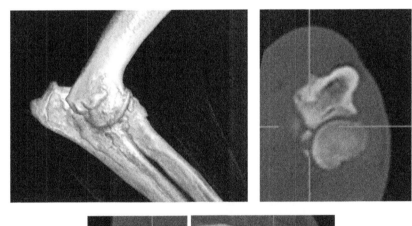

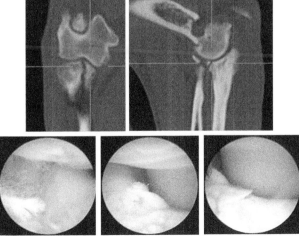

Arthroscopy: Synovitis, medial coronoid disease, and "kissing lesion."

9.2 Shoulder Tendinopathy

Case #2

CC: Left thoracic lameness, 3 months' duration
Age: Middle (5 years old)
Size: Large (28.0 kg), German Short-Haired Pointer (SF)
Problem: Biceps brachii tendon rupture and synovitis

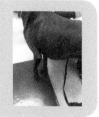

History

A 5-year-old spayed female German Short-Haired Pointer, presented for evaluation of persistent and worsening left forelimb lameness for three months.

- Her owner reported that she was running around outside, fell through the ice crust on top of the snow, and has been lame since that time. She expected the lameness to go away on its own, but over the last six weeks has noticed her signs are worsening and her energy level is lower.
- She was seen by her referring veterinarian, who took radiographs. She has not been prescribed any pain medications or anti-inflammatories.

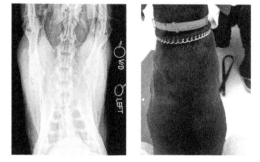

Physical Examination

- **Musculoskeletal**: Abnormal – significant lameness on front right limb, atrophy of muscles of proximal front right limb evident visually and on palpation (can see spine of scapula), well muscled on other limbs. Very painful on flexion and extension of the left shoulder joint. Also shows pain on palpation of left axilla or at the biceps tendon insertion point.

Diagnostic Tests, Radiology/CT Report

- The arthropathy is consistent with severe chronic degenerative joint disease characterized by severe mineralization of – or of the joint capsule surrounding – the proximal tendon of the biceps brachii muscle, and severe left-shoulder osteoarthrosis. Lameness is attributed to this finding, which is probably due to previous trauma.
- The results of this evaluation are negative for a malignant bone neoplasm.

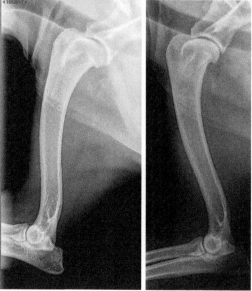

(Left)   (Right)

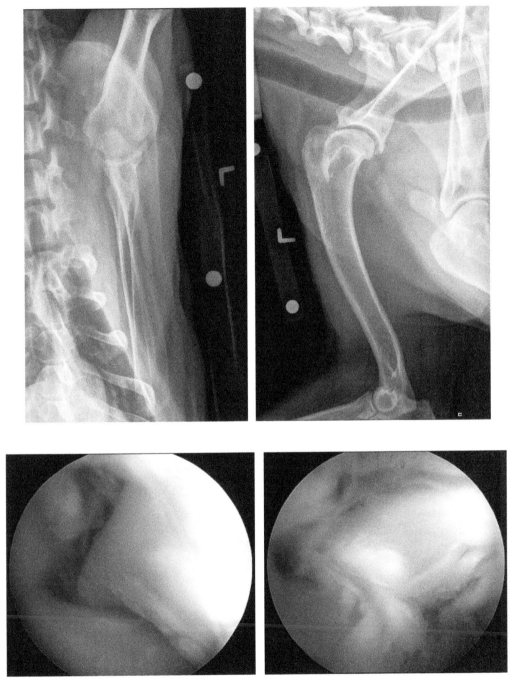

Arthroscopy: Partial rupture of biceps tendon and synovitis.

9.3 Shoulder Luxation in Small Dogs

Case #3

CC: Right thoracic limb lameness
Age: Old (9 years old)
Size: Small (2.4 kg), Yorkshire Terrier (FS)
Problem: Atraumatic medial shoulder luxation

Video 9.2 Thoracic limb lameness (shoulder luxation).

History

A 9-year-old female spayed Yorkshire Terrier presented for right forelimb lameness.

- About two months ago, she was non-weight bearing on the right front leg with no obvious pain. A shoulder luxation was diagnosed by the referring veterinarian.
- After 1–2 weeks of this onset, the right front leg was weight bearing again, but still seemed sensitive.
- There was no history of trauma, but she has a tendency of jumping off furniture.
- She has a previous history of a luxated right patella 1–2 years ago, which was treated surgically.

Physical Examination

- Grade 2/5 right thoracic limb lameness.
- Right thoracic limb: decreased shoulder extension, crepitus on range of motion; not overtly luxated at this time. Elbow held mildly abducted. Elbow, carpus, digits, and long bones palpate normally.
- Left thoracic limb: shoulder, elbow, carpus, digits, and long bones palpate normally; elbow held mildly abducted.
- Pelvic limbs: Bilateral grade 2–3 medial patellar luxation; suture palpable on lateral surface of right stifle, consistent with previous surgery. Otherwise, hips, stifles, tarsi, digits, and long bones palpate normally.

Diagnostic Tests, Radiology/CT Report

- The right shoulder joint is dislocated in some views, with the humeral head located medial to the glenoid cavity and with mild proximal displacement (overriding).
- Right shoulder dislocation with moderate displacement.
- Right thoracic limb lameness is attributed to shoulder dislocation. The results of this examination are negative for fracture.

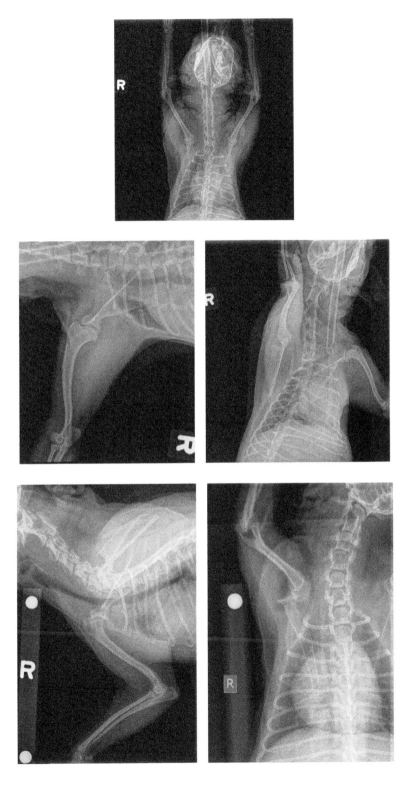

Case #4

CC: Right thoracic limb lameness
Age: Old (11 years old)
Size: Small (1.0 kg), Toy Poodle (NM)
Problem: Atraumatic medial shoulder luxation

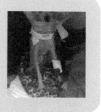

History

An 11-year-old male castrated Toy Poodle presented for acute onset of non-weight bearing on right front limb; no trauma was observed.

- He was evaluated by his primary care veterinarian, who prescribed analgesics and rest. He has not shown any improvement since the initial injury.
- Bloodwork was performed most recently by his primary veterinarian and revealed anemia (Hct 35.9), neutrophilia, and monocytosis consistent with an infection, and an elevated BUN (29) indicating prerenal azotemia.
- He received Metacam and tramadol and developed explosive diarrhea; no blood was seen in it.
- He is urinating and defecating normally at this time, and is not coughing, sneezing, or vomiting.

Physical Examination

- Ambulatory x3. Holds right forelimb in flexed position. Luxated right shoulder joint. No patellar luxation, stifles not thickened. Complete ortho exam not performed.

Diagnostic Tests, Radiology/CT Report

- Acute shoulder luxation, right.
- Recent dental extractions, mandible.
- Questionable left cardiomegaly.
- Conclusion: Lameness is attributed to the right shoulder luxation.

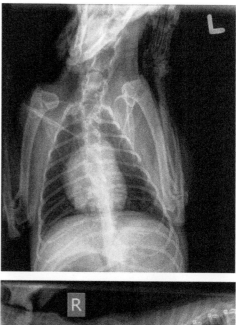

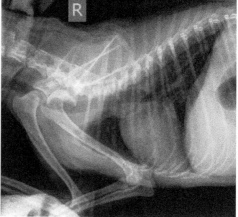

9.4 Carpal Hyperextension

Case #5

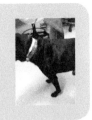

CC: Thoracic limb lameness for four months after injury
Age: Mature (7 years old)
Size: Large (35.5 kg), Labrador Retriever (SF)
Problem: Traumatic carpal hyperextension

Video 9.3 Thoracic limb lameness (carpal hyperextension).

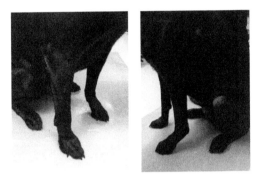

History

A 7-year-old spayed female Labrador Retriever presented for a left thoracic limb lameness for over four months.

- Four months ago, she jumped down from a height.
- Radiographs revealed no abnormality.
- Persistent lameness since. Getting worse.

Physical Examination

- Severe lameness on left front, dropped carpal joint. No pain on palpation. No other abnormalities.

Diagnostic Tests, Radiology/CT Report

- Lameness and carpal swelling are attributed to hyperextension injury (accessoriometacarpal, palmer intercarpal ligament ruptures) and subluxation.

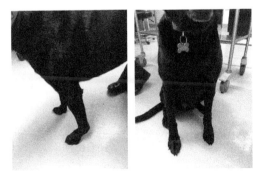

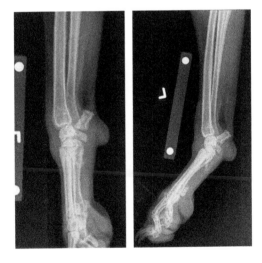

Case #6

CC: Thoracic limb lameness
Age: Mature (5 years old)
Size: Large (29.2 kg), Siberian Husky (NM)
Problem: Traumatic carpal hyperextension, medial collateral injury

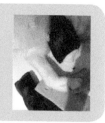

History

A 5-year-old male neutered Siberian Husky presented to the emergency service for acute onset of left front limb.

- Three days ago, the owner was on a hike and he ran up a hill out of site for a few moments. Owner noticed him limping and non-weight bearing on his left forelimb as he walked down the hill. Owner immediately carried him to the car and took him to a veterinary practice, where they took radiographs.
- He had significant soft tissue swelling of his left forelimb, so the veterinarian said to wait on wrapping and splinting his leg. His swelling significantly decreased overnight and the owner brought him back to have his leg wrapped and a splint placed. He was prescribed a pain medication, Deramaxx (75 mg).

Physical Examination

- **Musculoskeletal**: Abnormal – ambulatory x3, non-weight bearing on left forelimb, normal range of motion (ROM) x3; left forelimb splinted; no back pain; normal ROM of cervical spine; full orthopedic exam not performed.

Diagnostic Tests, Radiology/CT Report

- Lameness and carpal swelling are attributed to subluxation (medial collateral ligament, palmar intercarpal ligament ruptures).

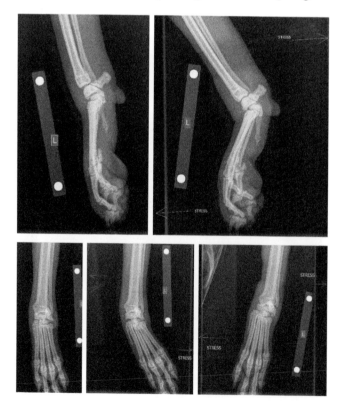

9.5 Neoplasia

Case #7

CC: Left thoracic limb lameness, chronic (for six months)
Age: Mature (8 years old)
Size: Large (30.2 kg), Irish Setter (NM)
Problem: Brachial plexus peripheral nerve sheath tumor

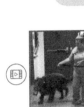

Video 9.4 Thoracic limb lameness (neoplasia).

History

An 8-year-old male castrated Irish Setter presented for a six-month history of left front-limb lameness.

- Six months ago, the lameness started acutely in the winter time after his left front limb fell heavy into some deep snow.
- Five months ago, radiographs were taken at the referring veterinarian, which revealed no abnormalities.
- Over the past few months, he has gotten progressively more painful and lame in the left front. He will tend to hold the limb up and out.

- He is currently on meloxicam (65 pounds dose once daily), tramadol (125 mg as needed for pain), and chondroitin/glucosamine supplement.
- No other health concerns were noted by the owners. He is eating, drinking, urinating, and defecating normally.

Physical Examination

- **Musculoskeletal**: Abnormal – severe muscle atrophy of the left front limb. Pain on palpation of the proximal left humerus. Ambulatory x4 with head bob and limping. Crepitus noted in the left carpus.

Diagnostic Tests, Radiology/CT Report

- Likely incidental interosseous enthesopathy vs. radioulnar ischemic necrosis, left antebrachium.
- Conclusion: A definitive cause for severe lameness is not determined during this evaluation. The results are negative for aggressive bone lesion (i.e., osteosarcoma) and bone fracture.

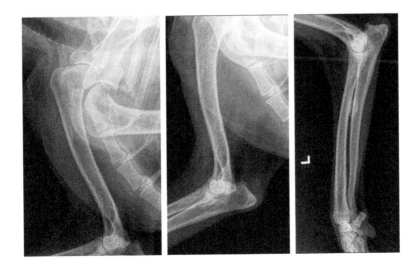

Ultrasound

- Moderate diffuse atrophy, left triceps.
- Conclusion: Moderate atrophy of the left triceps muscle is attributed to the cause of left thoracic limb lameness, for which the definitive etiology is not determined. The results of this evaluation are negative for rupture of the triceps muscle and rupture and avulsion of the triceps tendon.

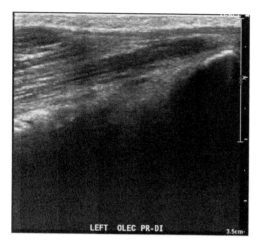

Magnetic Resonance Imaging (MRI)

- Extensive neuropathy, left brachial plexus.
- Moderate, diffuse muscle atrophy, left thoracic limb.
- Conclusion: The MRI appearance and extensive nature of the lesion in the left brachial plexus are suggestive that this is a neoplastic lesion with a peripheral nerve sheath tumor prioritized. Granulomatous neuritis of traumatic or inflammatory cause cannot be excluded. The diffuse muscle atrophy is consistent with the extensive nature, involving the distal branches of the C6–T2 nerves.

Biopsy/Histopathology

- Histologic features are consistent with malignant peripheral nerve sheath tumor.

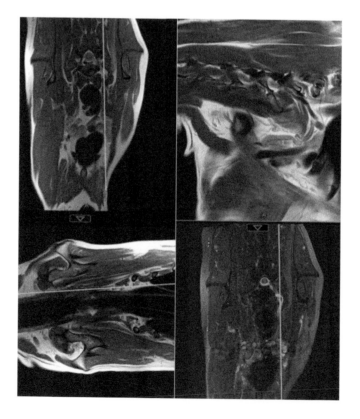

Case #8

CC: Right thoracic limb lameness
Age: Mature (3 years old)
Size: Large (27.0 kg), Pitbull Terrier mix (FS)
Problem: Proximal humeral/shoulder sarcoma

Video 9.5 Thoracic limb lameness (neoplasia).

Video 9.6 Thoracic limb lameness (view from behind) (neoplasia).

History

An approximately 3-year-old female spayed Staffordshire Terrier mix presented for evaluation of a two-week history of right forelimb lameness.

- Approximately two weeks ago, she was seen to be fighting with the neighbor dogs through the fence, although she reportedly did not make physical contact with them. She was seen digging up shrubs, bushes, and trying to get through the fence.
- After this episode, her owners noted that she was limping slightly on her right forelimb and by the next morning the lameness had progressed. They presented to the referring veterinarian the next morning for evaluation. Radiographs were taken and a physical exam was performed, which revealed significant right forelimb pain but no other abnormalities.
- She was started on carprofen, but it did not seem to help and she was noted to have increased urination while taking it, so it was discontinued.

- One week later the lameness was still present, so she was taken back to the referring veterinarian for repeat radiographs, which again revealed no obvious fractures or injuries to the joint. Tramadol was started, which the owners do not think made a difference.
- Approximately two days ago, she became acutely more painful and non-weight bearing, although there was no inciting incident witnessed that could explain the sudden progression of her clinical signs.
- She is crated when the owners are not at home, but does wrestle with her housemate. Since then, she has been lethargic, anorexic, has been drinking less, and has not defecated in the past 24 hours.
- Aside from tramadol (50 mg orally twice a day), she is not on any other medications or preventatives. The owners do not know her history prior to adopting her from the shelter approximately four months ago, but she is up to date on all vaccines. Prior to this incident, she has been healthy and very active while the owners have had her.

Physical Examination

- **Musculoskeletal**: Abnormal – all limbs within normal limits except right forelimb, which revealed severe pain on elbow extension, shoulder extension, and shoulder abduction in addition to moderate atrophy of the muscles of her right forelimb; no crepitus or effusion were noted on the right forelimb, but palpation and movement of the brachium and shoulder resulted in severe pain.
- **Nervous system**: Abnormal – mentation normal.

- Posture: Non-weight bearing on the right thoracic limb, and holding it in flexion.
- Mental status: Bright, alert, and responsive (BAR).
- Attitude/posture: Non-weight bearing on the right thoracic limb, and holding it in flexion.
- Conformation/muscularity: Normal apart from right thoracic limb, which had generalized muscle atrophy (especially biceps muscle).
- Gait: Walking well on the other three limbs with occasional placement and tentative weight bearing on the right thoracic limb.
- Cranial nerves: Normal.
- Proprioception: Unable to perform paw placement or hopping on right forelimb. Normal on the other three limbs.

- Spinal reflexes: Normal apart from right thoracic limb, which had absent withdrawal.
- Nociception: Severe pain on palpation of right forelimb.
- Neurolocalization: Right radial nerve/brachial plexus.

Diagnostic Tests, Radiology/CT Report

- Clinically normal thoracic radiographs.
- Monostotic aggressive bone lesion, right humerus.

Biopsy/Histopathology

- Histologic features are consistent with poorly differentiated sarcoma.

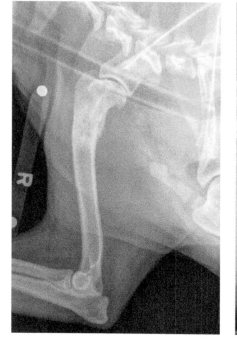

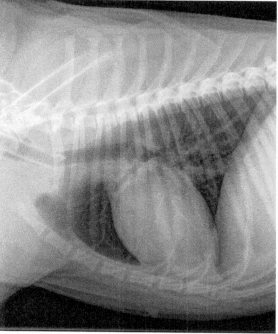

9.6 Immune-Mediated Poly-arthropathy

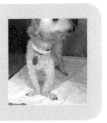

Case #9

CC: Bilateral carpal laxity
Age: Old (13 years old)
Size: Small (2.8 kg), Miniature Poodle
Problem: Immune-mediated poly-arthropathy (IMPA): erosive

History

An approximately 13-year-old female spayed Miniature Poodle presented for evaluation of bilateral carpal hyperextension and valgus.

- About six months ago, her owner started to notice her walking with her carpi hyperextended.
- This progressed over the next few months, and at about three months ago she started walking on her carpi.
- She was brought to her primary vet at this time – her owner was told that her carpal ligaments were stretched out. She was started on Deramaxx 12 mg once daily, and her owners believe that has helped with her comfort.

- In the last month, her carpi have continued to get even worse, and began to turn out (carpal valgus).
- She does not try to move around much, and has completely stopped running or jumping.
- She has maintained a good appetite, and has not had any other systemic signs of illness (coughing, sneezing, vomiting, or diarrhea).

Physical Examination

- **Musculoskeletal**: Abnormal – minimally ambulatory, bears weight on carpi bilaterally, carpi are hyperextended and mani are laterally deviated, carpi have severe crepitus and laxity, no pain; stifles: mild effusion bilaterally, crepitus, medially luxating patellas (grade 2) pin; hips: pain on extension, crepitus.

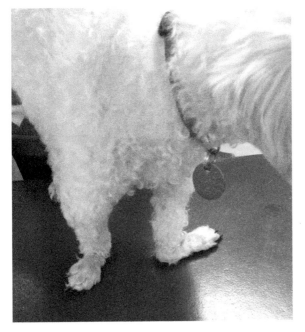

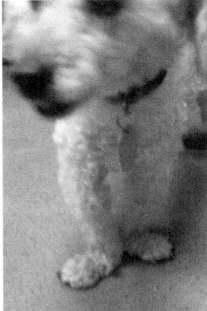

Diagnostic Tests, Radiology/CT Report

- Severe, erosive poly-arthropathy with subluxation and carpal valgus, bilateral carpi.
- Conclusion: Bilateral carpal laxity is attributed to the erosive poly-arthropathy with a

primary differential diagnosis of noninfectious polyarthritis (e.g., canine rheumatoid arthritis, immune-mediated arthritis).

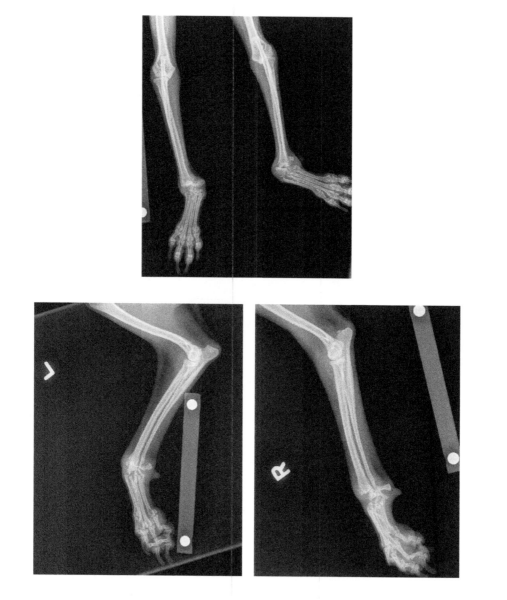

The videos are available for this chapter on www.wiley.com/go/hayashi/lameness.

10

Pelvic Limb Lameness in Young Dogs

10.1 Medial Patellar Luxation

> **Case #1**
>
> **Chief Complaint (CC)**: Bilateral hind limb gait abnormality (worse on the left)
> **Age**: Young (onset at 6 months old)
> **Size**: Small (2.2 kg at 7 months old), Toy Poodle mix (SF)
> **Problem**: Bilateral medial patellar luxation (grades 2–3)

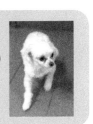

Video 10.1 Pelvic limb lameness (medial patellar luxation).

History

A 1.5-year-old female spayed mixed-breed dog presented for evaluation of a "funny," "cowboy-like" gait since an acute injury to her hindlimbs after jumping off the couch.

- She occasionally walks with the left leg off the ground.
- She was diagnosed with 3/4 patellar luxation in both hindlimbs and prescribed carprofen, which helped short term, but the owners believe her gait is getting worse and would like to pursue further treatment.

Physical Examination

- **Musculoskeletal**: Abnormal – atrophy of both hindlimb muscles, marked medial rotation of the tibia, grade 3/4 medial luxating patellas. Caudal cervical neck pain.
- **Nervous system**: Normal – normal proprioception.

Diagnostic Tests, Radiology/Computed Tomography (CT) Report

- Questionable intracapsular swelling, bilateral stifles.
- Conclusions: Stifle swelling is questionable, as the finding is mild and may be normal variation in a young dog. However, if real, it is attributed to clinical diagnosis of patellar luxation. Lucencies in the tibial tuberosity may be due to incomplete closure/remodeling of tibial apophyses in this skeletally immature dog, or possible retained cartilage, which has been associated with patellar luxation in dogs.

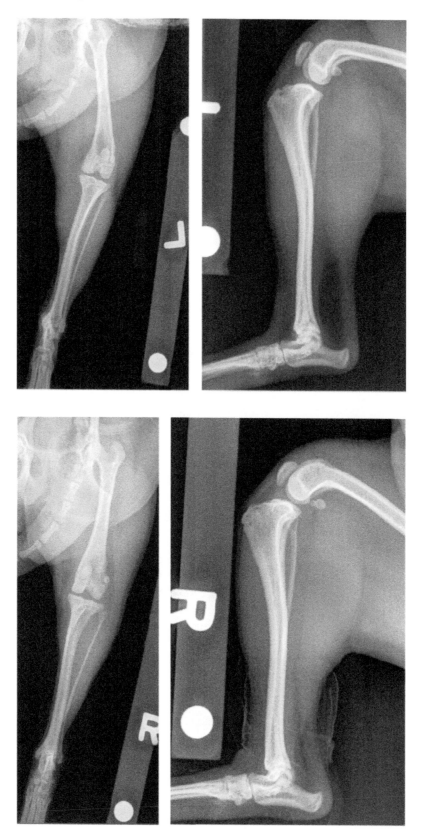

Case #2

CC: Bilateral hindlimb lameness and deformity
Age: Young (onset at 2 months old, presented at 3 months old)
Size: Small (3.3 kg), Shetland Sheepdog (F)
Problem: Bilateral medial patellar luxation (grade 4) and femoral and tibial deformities

Video 10.2a Pelvic limb lameness/deformity (medial patellar luxation).

Video 10.2b Pelvic limb lameness/deformity (medial patellar luxation).

History

A 3-month-old Shetland Sheepdog presented for bilateral hindlimb lameness.

- She was adopted three weeks ago, and the owner was told that she had tight tendons.
- She went to her primary care veterinarian 10 days ago because her gait had not improved, where physical exam and radiographs confirmed bilateral grade 4/4 medial patellar luxation.
- She is playing, and is not painful. She has been taking Cosequin daily. She is otherwise systemically healthy with no coughing/sneezing/vomiting/diarrhea (c/s/v/d) noted.

Physical Examination

- **Musculoskeletal**: Ambulatory x4, kyphotic posture, stifles held in flexion bilaterally, outward rotation of femurs bilaterally when walking, limited extension of stifles bilaterally, bilateral grade 4/4 medial patellar luxation, bilateral hypoplastic patella, no long bone pain or joint effusion.
- **Nervous system**: Appropriate mentation, cranial nerves within normal limits, full neuro exam not performed.

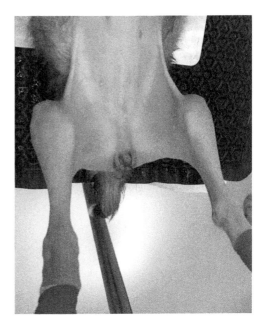

Diagnostic Tests, Radiology/CT Report

- Moderate bilateral rotational pelvic limb deformity.
- Severe bilateral medial patellar luxation with hypoplastic femoral trochlear groove.
- Incidental polydactyly, bilateral pelvic limbs.

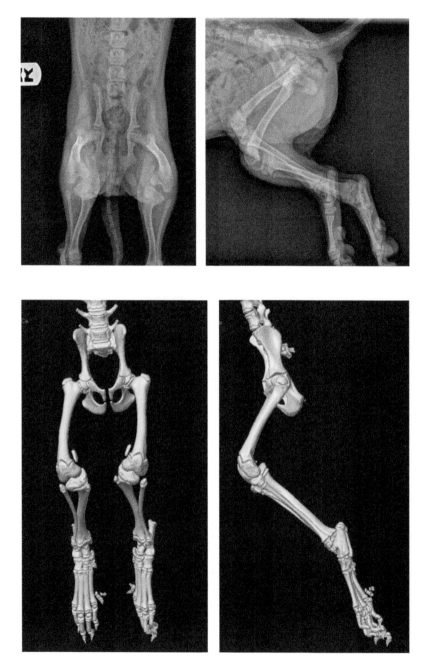

Case #3

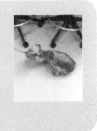

CC: Bilateral hindlimb lameness and deformity
Age: Young (onset about 3 months old, presented at 9 months old)
Size: Small (3.5 kg), Yorkshire Terrier (NM)
Problem: Bilateral medial patellar luxation (grade 4) and femoral and tibial deformities

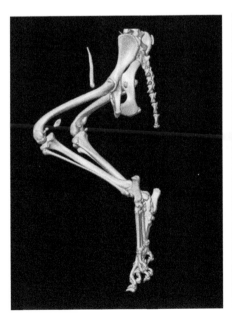

Video 10.3 Pelvic limb lameness/deformity (medial patellar luxation).

History

A 9-month-old male castrated Yorkshire Terrier presented for severe bilateral hindlimb lameness.

- Five months ago he was found in Mississippi, running along a busy highway with his litter mate after being thrown out of a car.
- Three months ago he was rescued by his current owner, and has had gait abnormalities since she got him. He is sometimes painful at night and after long periods of activity.

- He has a good activity level and is otherwise systemically healthy.

Physical Examination

- **Musculoskeletal**: Kyphotic posture. Stifles held in flexion bilaterally, decreased range of motion and pain on extension of stifles. Grade 4/4 bilateral medial luxation of patellas. Slightly decreased range of motion of hocks bilaterally. Minimal weight bearing of hindlimbs bilaterally, offloading of hindlimbs. Outward rotation of elbows bilaterally.
- **Nervous system**: Palpebral reflexes and menace response intact bilaterally, full neuro exam not performed.

Diagnostic Tests, Radiology/CT Report

- Severe bilateral medial patellar luxation with subsequent severe bilateral angular limb deformity.

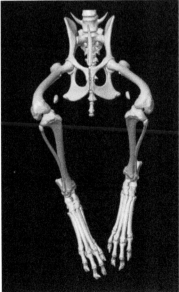

Case #4

CC: Bilateral hindlimb lameness, bowed-leg appearance
Age: Young (onset at 12 months old)
Size: Large (3.3 kg), Chihuahua (NM)
Problem: Bilateral medial patellar luxation (grade 3)

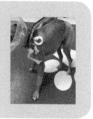

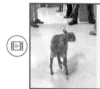

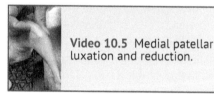

Video 10.4 Pelvic limb lameness (medial patellar luxation).

History

A 1.5-year-old male castrated Chihuahua presented for evaluation of bilateral gait abnormality and bowed-leg appearance.

- 5–6 months ago, his owners noticed that he developed a bow-legged stance.
- Since that time he has become progressively more lame in his left hindlimb and has stopped wanting to go up and down the stairs.
- He has no other medical conditions and has otherwise been a healthy dog. He was given Metacam occasionally for presumptive pain, but currently only receives Cosequin and Frontline.

Physical Examination

Medial patellar luxation, internal rotation of tibia, bilaterally.

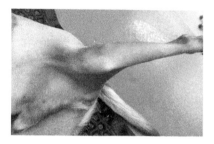

Video 10.5 Medial patellar luxation and reduction.

Diagnostic Tests, Radiology/CT Report

- Bilateral medial patellar luxation.
- Bilateral pelvic lameness is attributed to bilateral medial patellar luxation.

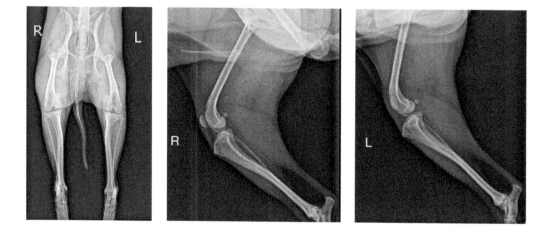

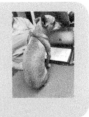

Case #5

CC: Bilateral hindlimb lameness
Age: Young (onset at 6 months old)
Size: Small (6.8 kg), Chihuahua mix (NM)
Problem: Bilateral medial patellar luxation (grade 2)

Video 10.6 Pelvic limb lameness (medial patellar luxation).

History

A 5-year-old male castrated Chihuahua mix was presented for evaluation of worsening of bilateral hindlimb lameness. He has had bilaterally luxating patella since he was adopted by his owner at around 6 months of age.

- The owner reports that this became a clinical issue at the beginning of this past summer. The patient's lameness substantially worsened once he began going on long walks and hikes; he couldn't go more than a mile without limping or wanting to sit down. The owner has decreased the amount of exercise since, which has helped the dog's lameness plateau. However, he appears stiff when he wakes up in the mornings and he starts to limp again if he goes on too long a walk. He has not received any medical management or physical therapy for this problem.

Physical Examination

- **Musculoskeletal**: Ambulatory x4. Intermittent bilateral hindlimb stiffness when walking (L apparently worse than R). Grade 2/4 bilateral medial patellar luxation. Mild asymmetry of proximal hindlimb musculature (L subjectively smaller than R). No cranial drawer or tibial thrust elicited in either hindlimb. No joint pain, effusion, or instability.
- **Nervous system**: Appropriate mentation. Menace intact both eyes (OU). Palpebral reflex present OU. Pupillary light reflex (PLR; direct and consensual) present OU. No ataxia. Complete neuro exam not performed.

Diagnostic Tests, Radiology/CT Report

- Mild bilateral medial patellar luxation.
- Mild left hip joint laxity.
- Transitional lumbosacral vertebra.
- Impression: The results of this evaluation are positive for bilateral medial patellar luxation. The left hip joint laxity may be associated with the unilateral articulation of transverse process of transitional lumbosacral vertebra, or alternatively may be artifactual secondary to mild pelvic rotation.

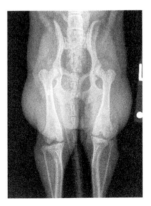

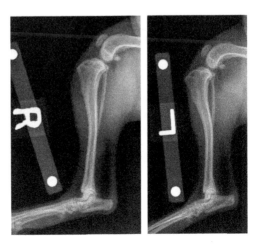

> **Case #6**
>
> **CC**: Bilateral hindlimb lameness, bow-legged appearance
> **Age**: Young (onset at 12 months old)
> **Size**: Small (6.8 kg), mix (SF)
> **Problem**: Bilateral medial patellar luxation (grade 3)

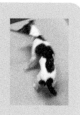

Video 10.7 Stiff gait (medial patellar luxation).

Video 10.8 Medial patellar luxation and reduction.

History

A 2-year-old female spayed terrier mix presented for an evaluation of her bilateral hindlimb gait abnormality. She was adopted approximately one year ago.

- Six months ago, it was noted that she began lifting her left leg and skipping, but did not appear painful at this time.
- Three months ago, she went to her primary care veterinarian for an annual examination, where it was discovered that both of her patellas were luxated.
- Her lameness is worse after she has been resting and appears to improve with activity.
- She is up to date on her vaccinations and is currently receiving Dasaquin and heartworm preventative.

Physical Examination

- **Musculoskeletal**: Abnormal – bilaterally symmetric musculature. No atrophy noted. No lameness appreciated. No pain on palpation of long bones. Grade 3/4 medial luxating patellas. Crepitus on reduction of the patellas.
- **Nervous system**: Normal – appropriate mentation, central nervous system (CNS) intact, no ataxia noted. Full examination not performed.

Diagnostic Tests, Radiology/CT Report

- Mild, bilateral stifle osteoarthrosis with mild stifle effusion (R>L).
- The changes are ascribed for the reported bilateral patellar luxation. Patellar luxation not identified radiographically.

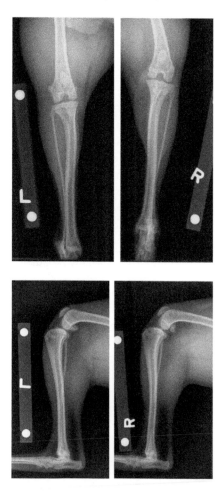

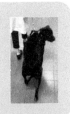

Case #7

CC: Bilateral hindlimb lameness
Age: Young (onset at 13 months old)
Size: Large (35.2 kg), mix (NM)
Problem: Bilateral medial patellar luxation (grade 2–3), stifle effusion

Video 10.9 Stiff gait (medial patellar luxation).

- **Nervous system**: Normal – full neuro exam not performed. Appropriate mentation. Cranial nerve reflexes intact: PLR, palpebral, menace, tongue, and jaw tone intact. No ataxia, normal conscious proprioception. Ambulatory x4. Lame on left hindlimb.

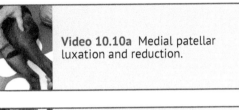

Video 10.10a Medial patellar luxation and reduction.

Video 10.10b Medial patellar luxation and reduction (spontaneous).

History

A 1.5-year-old castrated mixed dog presented for left hindlimb lameness.

- The process was gradual, but two months ago he started to become more visibly lame and pick up his leg.
- Owner reports no coughing, sneezing, vomiting, diarrhea, changes in urination or drinking. He is on Dasuquin (1 tablet once a day) and heartworm, flea, and tick preventatives.

Physical Examination

- **Musculoskeletal**: Abnormal – muscle atrophy in left hindlimb. Grade 3 patellar luxation in left hindlimb; grade 1 patellar luxation in right hindlimb. Offloading the left hindlimb and hyperextending the hock during standing. For the rest of the orthopedic exam, there was no obvious pain, fracture, effusion, or crepitus appreciated on exam, no pain on palpation of long bones or joint manipulation.

Diagnostic Tests, Radiology/CT Report

- Left luxating patella with mild to moderate osteoarthrosis, mild to moderate intracapsular swelling, and mild muscle atrophy.
- Mild right-stifle osteoarthrosis with mild intracapsular swelling.
- Mild bilateral hip enthesopathy.
- The radiographic signs are consistent with the history of left medially luxating patella.

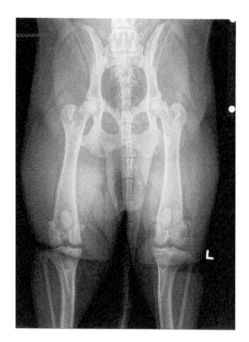

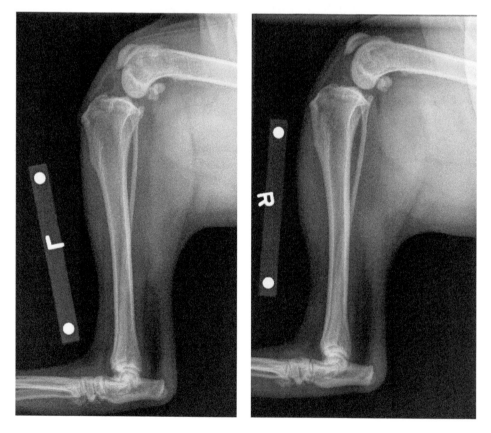

10.2 Lateral Patellar Luxation

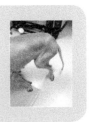

Case #8

CC: Bilateral hindlimb lameness for 10 months
Age: Young (onset at 6 months old, presented at 1 year 3 months old)
Size: Giant (60 kg), Great Dane (M)
Problem: Bilateral lateral patellar luxation (grade 4)

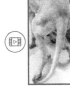

Video 10.11 Abnormal posture (lateral patellar luxation/deformity).

History

A nearly 16-month-old intact Great Dane presented for evaluation of a non-weight-bearing bilateral hindlimb lameness of 10 months' duration.

- At 6 months of age he had an acute episode of recumbency, hindlimb discomfort, and hyperthermia of one day's duration. Subsequently, he has repeated episodes of hindlimb discomfort that the owner reports occurring following times of rapid growth in stature.
- Immediately prior to these growth periods, he tends to display a more normal extension of his hindlimbs and will bear more weight on his foot pads. The owner reports that he has been seen by multiple veterinarians during this time with no definitive diagnosis or indication of what is causing his lameness.
- The owner performs massage on his hindlimbs daily and passive range of motion exercises. The patient has received chiropractic manipulations of his hind end as well as acupuncture sessions. Following acupuncture, he will ambulate and bear weight with significant improvement; however, the results last less than 24 hours.
- Suspecting hypertrophic osteopathy, he was administered a tapering dose of prednisone starting at 50 mg for a period of 7 weeks.

This was discontinued due to fear of muscle wasting from prolonged corticosteroid use and the owner reports that his level of hindlimb musculature has increased over the past couple months.

- Other relevant history includes that he was on a raw diet for his first six months, he had been vaccinated just prior to his six-month episode, and he has been switched to dry food due to a more appropriate calcium: phosphorus ratio and decreased protein content.

Physical Examination

- **Musculoskeletal**: Abnormal – on orthopedic examination he was non-weight bearing to toe-touching lame bilaterally in his pelvic limbs, with increased flexion at all joints and a knocked-knee confirmation. There was marked atrophy and contracture of both his quadriceps and sartorius muscles bilaterally, as well as atrophy of his gluteal and caudal/inner thigh muscles.
- There was decreased range of motion (most notable on extension) at the tarsus, stifle, and hip bilaterally, although no elicitation of pain response. Patellar and withdrawal reflexes were present bilaterally, but decreased due to the decreased range of motion. General proprioception was intact bilaterally.
- On stifle palpation there was diffuse soft tissue swelling and medial buttress bilaterally, along with presumed lateral displacement of the patellas bilaterally. A mild reaction was noted upon stifle manipulation.

- **Nervous system**: Normal – appropriate mentation; normal proprioception; intact menace/PLR/facial sensation; intact withdrawal and patellar reflexes.

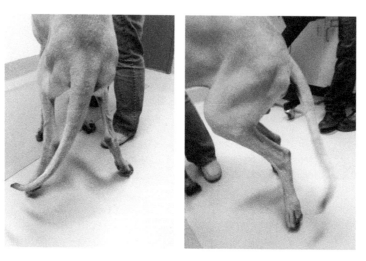

Diagnostic Tests, Radiology/CT Report

- Severe lateral patellar luxation and osteoarthrosis, both stifles.
- Moderate to severe malformation of the distal diaphysis and lateral condyle, both femurs.
- Severe muscle atrophy, thigh and crus muscles, both pelvic limbs.
- Conclusion: Hindlimb lameness is attributed to bilateral lateral patellar luxation and osteoarthrosis.

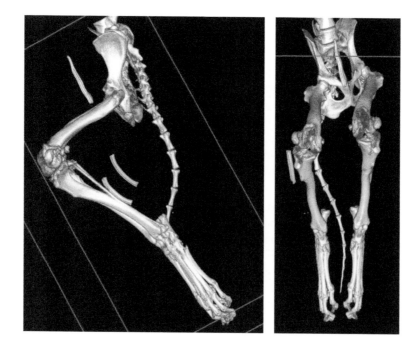

10.3 Hip Dysplasia

> ### Case #9
>
> **CC**: Bilateral hindlimb gait abnormality
> **Age**: Young (onset at 4 months old)
> **Size**: Large (24.4 kg at 13 months old), Boxer mix (SF)
> **Problem**: Bilateral hip dysplasia (mild)

Video 10.12 Stiff gait (hip dysplasia).

History

A 13-month-old female spayed Boxer mix presented for evaluation of chronic bilateral hindlimb lameness.

- About nine months ago (age about 4 months old) when she was adopted, she began displaying signs of having stiffness and pain when rising from lying down as well as limping and pain in both hips after activity.
- Additionally, since adoption, the owners have noticed her having hip instability, where she will splay her hind legs out and fall as well as cross her legs while walking.
- About a month ago (at 12 months old), she visited her local veterinarian and at this time radiographs were performed and she was diagnosed with severe bilateral hip dysplasia.
- At that time, she was prescribed carprofen and gabapentin.
- Since the time of her diagnosed hip dysplasia, she has gotten progressively more lame and painful.

Physical Examination

- **Musculoskeletal**: Abnormal – pain on terminal extension of bilateral coxofemoral joints (worse on left), with offloading of bilateral pelvic limbs when standing (worse on left); referred epaxial and iliopsoas pain; bilateral mild elbow joint effusion. The remainder of her orthopedic exam was normal.

- **Nervous system**: Normal – conscious proprioception (CP) normal; cranial nerves intact; full neurologic exam not performed.

Diagnostic Tests, Radiology/CT Report

- Moderate bilateral hip dysplasia with mild bilateral hip osteoarthrosis.
- Mild focal dystrophic mineralization, right semitendinosus muscle.
- Conclusion: The results of this evaluation are positive for bilateral hip dysplasia.

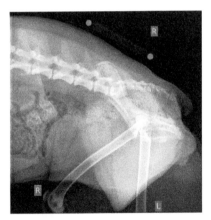

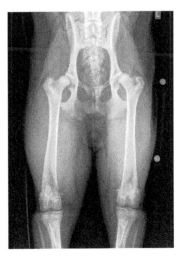

Case #10

CC: Bilateral hindlimb lameness
Age: Young (onset at 4 months old)
Size: Medium (16.1 kg at 12 months old), Australian Shepherd (M)
Problem: Bilateral hip dysplasia/subluxation (severe)

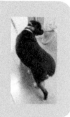

Video 10.13a Pelvic limb lameness/stiff gait (hip dysplasia).

Video 10.13b Pelvic limb lameness/stiff gait (hip dysplasia) (left side).

Video 10.13c Pelvic limb lameness/stiff gait (hip dysplasia) (right side).

History

A 1-year-old intact male Australian Shepherd presented for severe bilateral hindlimb lameness.

- His owners have had him since he was 4 months old.
- When he was a puppy they noticed he walked with an odd gait where he didn't want to extend his right hind leg.

Physical Examination

- **Musculoskeletal**: Abnormal – bilateral hip pain on extension, base-narrow stance behind, lameness more pronounced on the right side. Normal sit test.
- **Nervous system**: Normal – appropriate mentation, cranial nerve exam and peripheral reflexes within normal limits.

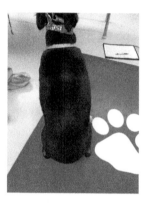

Diagnostic Tests, Radiology/CT Report

- Bilateral hip dislocation with moderate to severe degenerative joint disease (R>L).
- Bilateral disuse atrophy of the pelvic limbs.
- The pelvic limb lameness is attributed to severe hip dysplasia and associated degenerative joint disease.

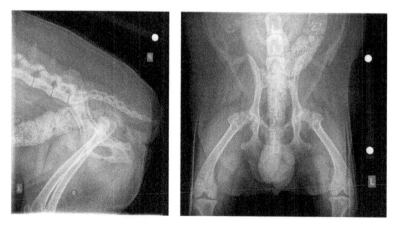

10.4 Femoral Head Necrosis (Legg–Calve–Perthes Disease) and Related Conditions

Case #11

CC: Right pelvic limb lameness
Age: Young (onset at 6 months old, presented at 11 months old)
Size: Small (3.6 kg), Yorkshire Terrier mix (NM)
Problem: Femoral head necrosis

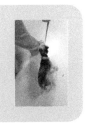

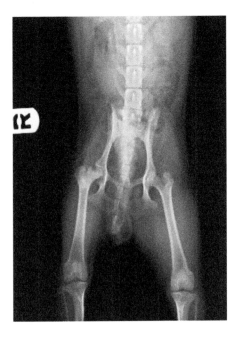

Video 10.14 Pelvic limb lameness (femoral head necrosis).

History

An 11-month-old male castrated Yorkie mix presented for evaluation of a right hindlimb lameness.

- Eight months ago (when he was 3 months old), he fell off the couch and seemed sore on his right hind leg, but the owner reported that this seemed to resolve.
- Six months ago, he fell off the couch again, and again acted sore on his right hind leg.
- He generally bears weight on his right hindlimb, but often limps or holds the leg up. The owner does not think that the patient's lameness has progressed since the incident, but it has stayed constant.
- He was prescribed five days of carprofen on two separate occasions for this lameness, and the owner does not think that the medication helped.
- He was recently neutered (~two weeks ago), and after that procedure he was given carprofen again, to no effect.
- Pelvic radiographs were taken at the time of his neuter and the owner reports that the veterinarian was concerned about "necrosis in his hip" based on the radiographs.
- He goes for daily short walks, but is generally sedentary.

Physical Examination

- **Musculoskeletal**: Grade 3/5 right pelvic limb lameness.
  - Right pelvic limb: painful on hip range of motion; no hip luxation palpable, and not overtly painful on direct pressure over greater trochanter. Stifle, patella, tarsus, digits, and long bones palpate normally.
  - Left pelvic limb: hip, stifle, patella, tarsus, digits, and long bones palpate normally.
- **Nervous system**: Appropriate mentation. No ataxia or proprioceptive deficits observed. Withdrawals normal in all limbs. Menace, palpebral reflex, and PLR intact. Full neurologic exam not performed.

Diagnostic Tests, Radiology/CT Report

- Moderate, patchy lysis, right femoral head and neck.
- Moderate right pelvic limb disuse muscle atrophy.

- The primary differential diagnosis for the radiographic changes is avascular necrosis of the femoral head and neck (Legg–Calve–Perthes disease).

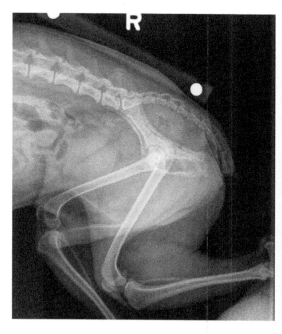

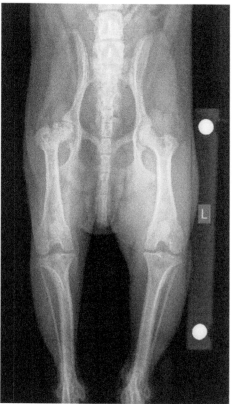

Case #12

CC: Right pelvic limb lameness
Age: Young (onset at 3 months old, presented at 10 months old)
Size: Small (4.1 kg), Yorkshire Terrier mix (NM)
Problem: Femoral head necrosis (suspect) or hip dysplasia/osteoarthritis

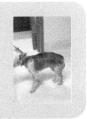

Video 10.15 Pelvic limb lameness (hip pain).

History

A 10-month-old castrated male Yorkie with an approximately seven-month history of non-weight-bearing lameness in his right hind leg.

- His owners think the onset of the lameness may have coincided with him jumping off the couch.
- He still likes to play and run with the Labrador Retriever that he lives with, and occasionally toe-touches on his right hindlimb, but otherwise does not use that leg.
- Four months ago, he was seen by his referring veterinarian, and prescribed Deramaxx for pain control.

- Based on radiographs obtained by the referring veterinarian, the diagnosis of hip dysplasia was made.

Physical Examination

- **Musculoskeletal**: Abnormal – 5/5 lame right hindlimb, non-weight bearing to toe-touching, walks and stands with limb completely flexed, resents palpation and extension of R hip, severe muscle atrophy R hindlimb, patellar tendons intact bilaterally, no crepitus in any other joints, no pain on vertebral palpation, no pain on tail manipulation.
- **Nervous system**: Normal – cranial nerves intact, general proprioception intact x4, full neuro exam not performed at this time.

Diagnostic Tests, Radiology/CT Report

Not available.

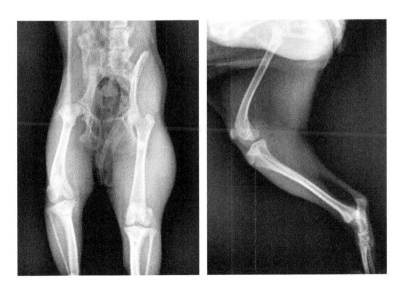

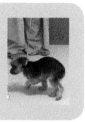

Case #13

CC: Bilateral pelvic limb lameness
Age: Young (onset at 7 months old, presented at 11 months old)
Size: Small (2.48 kg), Yorkshire Terrier (SF)
Problem: Bilateral Salter–Harris type 1 femoral capital physeal fractures

Video 10.16a Pelvic limb lameness/abnormal posture (hip pain).

Video 10.16b Pelvic limb lameness (hip pain).

History

An 11-month-old female spayed Yorkshire Terrier presented for evaluation of bilateral hindlimb lameness.

- Four months ago, she was first noted to be crossing her hindlimbs while walking.
- This progressed to the point where her gait was continuously abnormal when walking, she was periodically down on her hind end, and her hip seemed very painful when manipulated. Her left leg appeared worse than her right.
- Three months ago, she was seen by her primary veterinarian, who started her on carprofen. Bloodwork performed at that time was normal.
- Her condition has been stable since but has not improved. She remains on her carprofen once daily but is not on any other medications.
- She is otherwise healthy and still wants to be active.

Physical Examination

- **Musculoskeletal**: Abnormal – bilateral hindlimb lameness; forelimbs normal; normal tarsal and stifle joints; hips severely painful on flexion/extension.
- **Nervous system**: abnormal – appropriate mentation; ambulatory x4; cranial nerves intact; pain on palpation of lumbosacral spinal cord; no deficits noted; full neuro exam not performed.

Diagnostic Tests, Radiology/CT Report

- Bilateral chronic femoral capital physeal fracture – Salter–Harris type 1 with secondary bilateral moderate hip osteoarthrosis.
- Incidental, right anal sac emphysema.
- The changes in the proximal femurs are likely secondary to chronic, nonhealing fracture through both femoral proximal physes. A concurrent avascular necrosis of both femoral heads is possible and cannot be ruled out.

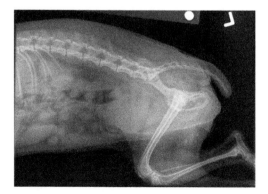

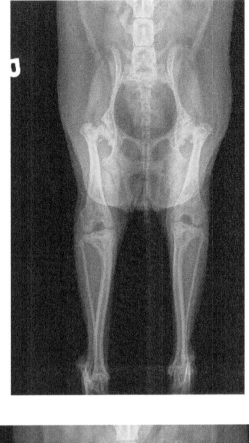

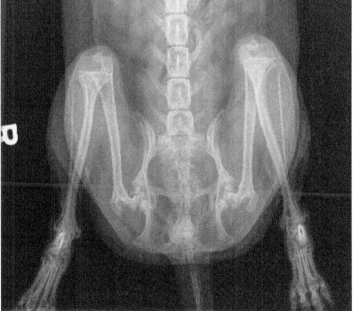

10.5   Tarsal/Stifle Osteochondritis Dissecans

> **Case #14**
>
> **CC**: Thoracic and pelvic limb lameness
> **Age**: Young (8 months old)
> **Size**: Large (29.4 kg at 8 months), Labrador Retriever (SF)
> **Problem**: Tarsal osteochondritis dissecans (OCD) and bilateral elbow dysplasia

Video 10.17 Pelvic limb lameness (tarsal OCD).

History

An 8-month-old, female spayed yellow Labrador Retriever presented for a chronic lameness.

- Three months ago, when she was about 5 months old, she first exhibited signs of pain and lameness. Her lameness would resolve after prolonged periods of rest, but would worsen after prolonged periods of activity/exercise.
- She was also noted to have a strange gait. Her chiropractor and veterinarian presumed the cause of her lameness to be elbow dysplasia; however, no diagnostic imaging was performed. Joint supplements were recommended.
- Two months ago, she jumped off a golf cart and yelped upon hurting her leg. Her lameness remained the same and did not worsen.

Physical Examination

- **Musculoskeletal**: Mild thickening of R/L tibiotarsal joints, no stifle effusion, normal coxofemoral joint manipulation.

Diagnostic Tests, Radiology/CT Report

- Bilateral OCD of the media trochlear ridge of the talus (L>>R).
- Mild right and moderate to severe left intracapsular swelling of the tarsocrural joint and effusion of the deep digital flexor (flexor halluces longus) tendon sheath.
- The clinical signs associated with the tarsi are attributed to the bilateral OCD and associated findings (intracapsular swelling, deep digital flexor tendon sheath effusion), worse in the left tarsus. The primary differential diagnosis for the tendon sheath effusion is synovitis or tenosynovitis.

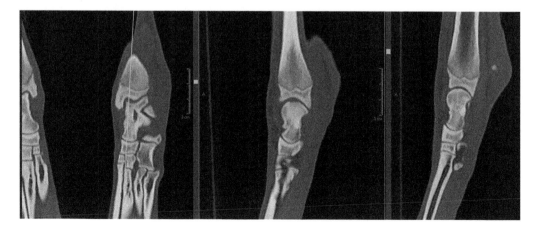

Case #15

CC: Left pelvic limb lameness
Age: Young (onset at 5 months old, presented at 8 months old)
Size: Large (23.5 kg at 8 month), Labrador Retriever (SF)
Problem: Tarsal OCD

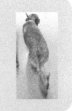

Video 10.18 Pelvic limb lameness (tarsal OCD).

Diagnostic Tests, Radiology/CT Report
- Large OCD lesion of the left talus with moderate tarsocrural effusion and mild osteoarthrosis.
- Normal bilateral elbow and right tarsus CT.

History
An 8-month-old female spayed Labrador Retriever presented for left hindlimb lameness.

- Three months ago, she first developed a left pelvic limb lameness, which had gradually progressed from occasional non-weight-bearing lameness to daily episodes of difficulty getting up and non-weight-bearing lameness of the left hindlimb.
- Radiographs revealed a small bone fragment at the medial aspect of the left talus. No medications were administered. She has otherwise been a healthy dog.

Physical Examination
- **Musculoskeletal**: Abnormal – ambulatory x4. Left hock was swollen, with moderate to severe effusion easily palpated. Pain elicited on palpation of the left hock and both elbow joints.
- **Nervous system**: Mentation appears normal. No cranial nerve deficits. Palpebral and menace reflexes intact.

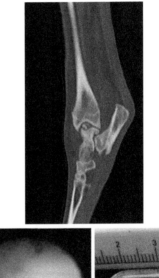

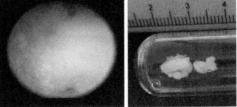

Arthroscopy: Tarsal OCD and removed OCD flap.

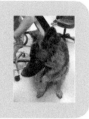

Case #16

CC: Bilateral pelvic limb lameness
Age: Young (onset at 4 months old, presented at 7 months old)
Size: Large (33 kg at 8 months old), German Shepherd (M)
Problem: Stifle OCD (bilateral), Lumbo-sacral disease suspected.

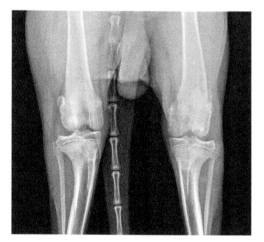

Video 10.19 Pelvic limb lameness/gait abnormality (stifle OCD, LS disease).

History

A 7-month-old male intact German Shepherd dog presented for trouble walking (seems painful in the rear legs).

- Since he was 4 months old, he has had an odd gait. Gait has become progressively worse, and the tops of his nails are worn.
- He no longer tries to jump into the truck, and is hesitant to go up stairs. He occasionally yelps when the owner manipulates his back legs or when he is picked up to place on a scale.
- He was given Rimadyl for one week, but the owners did not see any significant change or improvement. He is not currently on Rimadyl.

Physical Examination

- **Musculoskeletal**: Ambulatory x4; unofficial ortho consult obtained, pain on manipulation of stifles bilaterally (more so on extension of left stifle). Worn toe nails in hind paws.
- **Neurologic**: Sunken hind end. Low tail carriage. Pain on lumbosacral palpation. Scuffing on hindlimbs. Normal CP and withdrawals. Normal cranial nerves.

Diagnostic Tests, Radiology/CT Report

- Bilateral OCD of the lateral femoral condyle.

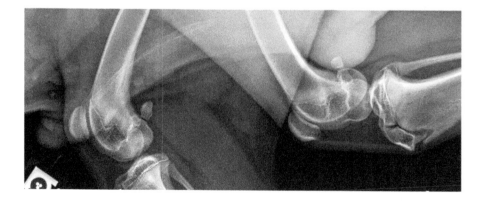

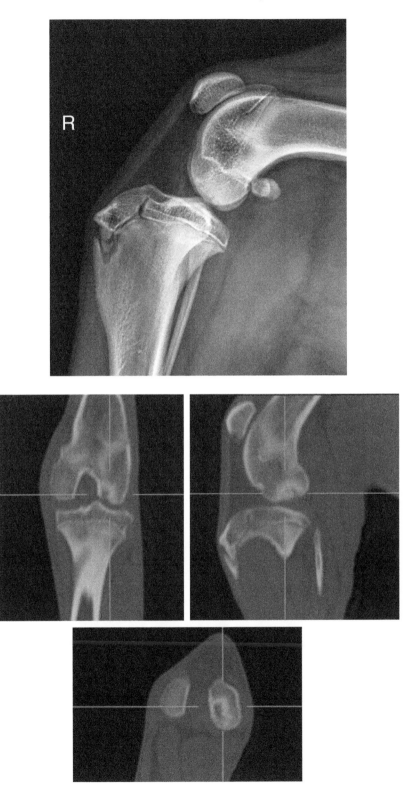

10.6 Physeal Fractures, Avulsion Fractures

Case #17

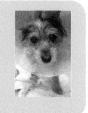

CC: Right pelvic limb lameness, acute onset after a minor trauma
Age: Young (6 months old)
Size: Small (1.9 kg at 6 months old), Yorkie-Poo mix (SF)
Problem: Tibial tuberosity avulsion fracture

History
A 6-month-old female spayed Yorkie-Poo presented for acute onset of right pelvis limb lameness.

- Her owner noticed non-weight bearing on her right hindlimb. The owner did not witness or hear any incident.
- She is otherwise a happy and healthy puppy with no previous medical issues and no medication at home.

Physical Examination
- **Musculoskeletal**: Ambulatory x4, toe-touching on right hindlimb, right stifle: joint distension and pain. No other joint abnormalities. No pain with long bone palpation, no pain with flexion/extension of forelimb and left hindlimb – did not perform full extension/flexion of right hindlimb.
- **Nervous system**: Normal – normal mentation, gait, attitude, posture. Normal CNS evaluation. Normal postural reactions and reflexes – patellar not performed.

Diagnostic Tests, Radiology/CT Report
- Acute traumatic tibial tuberosity avulsion fracture, right.

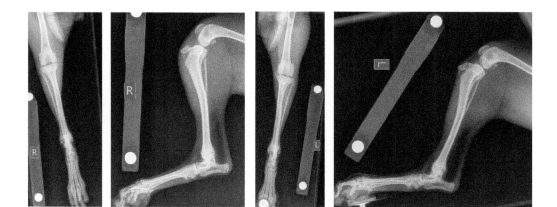

Case #18

CC: Left pelvic limb lameness, acute onset after a minor trauma
Age: Young (3.5 months old)
Size: Large (11.0 kg at 3.5 months old), Goldendoodle (F)
Problem: Long digital tendon avulsion fracture

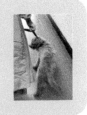

Video 10.20 Pelvic limb lameness (LDE avulsion).

History

A 14-week-old intact female Goldendoodle presented for evaluation of her left hindlimb lameness.

- About two weeks ago, she was being walked by the owner on a leash and the neighbor's two dogs, who were also being walked on leashes, came up to greet. All of the dogs got tangled up in one another and the owner heard her cry out and she was acutely non-weight bearing on her left hindlimb.
- She was brought to an emergency clinic that day, where radiographs were not taken and she was sent home on gabapentin (100 mg twice daily).
- She did not improve much with gabapentin alone and was taken to her primary vet four days later. Radiographs were obtained that revealed a small fragment of bone within her left stifle joint. She was then taken to a specialty hospital for an evaluation with their surgical service. They also prescribed carprofen (25 mg twice daily), which seemed to help a little, but she was still limping.
- As the three weeks passed from initial injury to presentation today, she has been bearing

more weight on that limb and jumps and puts weight on both hindlimbs normally according to the owner. She has been crate rested as much as possible given her activity level.

Physical Examination

- **Musculoskeletal**: Abnormal – severely atrophied left hind quadriceps and hamstring musculature, ambulatory x4 with mild to moderate lameness at the walk and trot, always weight bearing. Pain on manipulation of the left stifle joint with positive cranial drawer (thrust not performed). No stifle effusion appreciated bilaterally. No palpable long bone pain; remainder of ortho examination within normal limits (WNL).
- **Nervous system:** Normal – full neuro exam not performed. Appropriate mentation. Cranial nerve reflexes intact: PLR, palpebral, menace, tongue, gag, and jaw tone intact. Reflexes not assessed. No ataxia, normal conscious proprioception. Ambulatory x4.

Diagnostic Tests, Radiology/CT Report

- Mineral bodies, cranio-lateral stifle joint.
- Mild stifle joint effusion.
- The described mineral bodies are most consistent with avulsion fracture fragments of the proximal attachment of the long digital extensor tendon, and are less likely to be dystrophic mineralization of the tendon.

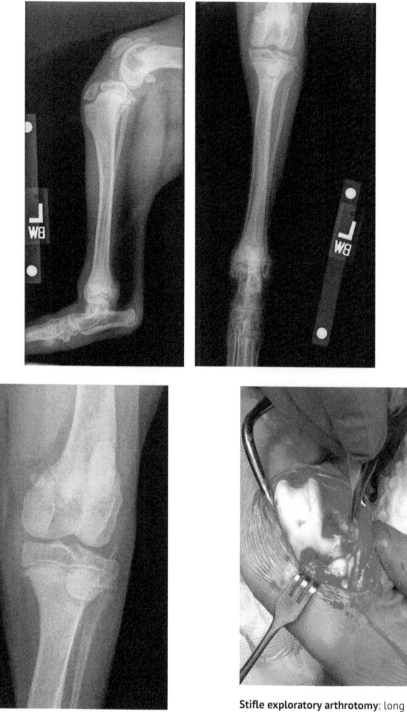

Stifle exploratory arthrotomy: long digital tendon avulsion fracture.

The videos are available for this chapter on www.wiley.com/go/hayashi/lameness.

11

Pelvic Limb Lameness in Mature Dogs

11.1 Cruciate Disease

Case #1

Chief Complaint (CC): Chronic bilateral hindlimb lameness
Age: Mature (5 years old)
Size: Large (34.6 kg), Pitbull mixed (SF)
Problem: Bilateral cranial cruciate ligament (CCL) disease (complete CCL rupture) with torn meniscus

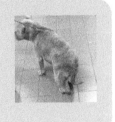

Video 11.1 Pelvic limb lameness (CCLD).

History
A 5-year-old female spayed mixed-breed dog presented for chronic history of bilateral hindlimb lameness from a shelter (no relevant history available).

Physical Examination
- **Musculoskeletal**: Abnormal – joint swelling/effusion bilaterally on the pelvic limb upon palpation. Questionable drawer/thrust. Pain on stifle palpation bilaterally. No hip pain.

- **Nervous system**: Normal – bright, alert and responsive (BAR). Central nervous system (CNS) intact. Normal conscious proprioception (CP) x4.

Diagnostic Tests, Radiology/Computed Tomography (CT) Report
- The left stifle joint has a moderate increased fluid opacity that distends the joint capsule cranially and caudally, and a low number of small periarticular osteophytes. The tibial condyles are cranially displaced relative to the femoral condyles. The soft tissues medial to the stifle joint are mildly thick (medial buttress). The crural muscles are mildly small.
- The right stifle joint has a moderately increased fluid opacity that distends the joint capsule cranially and caudally and a

small number of medium-sized periarticular osteophytes. The tibial condyles are cranially displaced relative to the femoral condyles. The soft tissues medial to the stifle joint are mildly thick (medial buttress). The crural muscles are mildly small.

- Within the soft tissues proximal to the calcaneal tuber, associated with the calcaneal tendon, there is a small amount of smoothly margined mineralization.

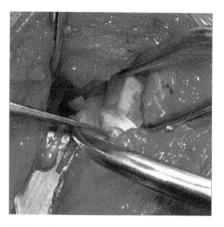

Stifle exploratory arthrotomy: CCL rupture and meniscal tear.

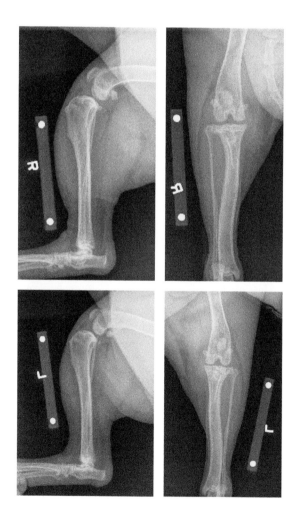

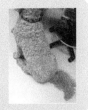

Case #2

CC: Left hindlimb lameness, 6 months' duration
Age: Mature (4 years and 3 months old)
Size: Large (26.4), mixed (NM)
Problem: Bilateral CCL disease (partial, chronic) intact meniscus

History

A 4-year-old male castrated mixed-breed canine presented for chronic history of left hindlimb lameness that started six months ago.

- Six months ago, the lameness started after he jumped into an empty pool. He was fine, but became painful thereafter.
- He has since progressively gotten worse.
- Three months ago, he was taken to his referring veterinarian and radiographs were taken; he was diagnosed with a CCL tear.
- The owner reports that he is painful when sitting and the lameness on the left hindlimb worsens with increased activity. He was on pain medications (the owner is unsure of the name) and he was on and off it.
- He is currently not on any medications aside from the preventatives (flea and tick).

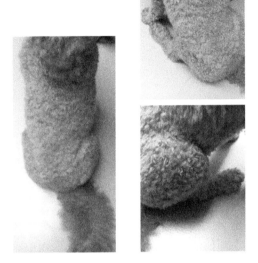

Physical Examination

- **Musculoskeletal**: Abnormal – slight left pelvic limb weight-bearing lameness. Mild cranial drawer with negative cranial tibial thrust on the left pelvic limb. No evidence of joint effusion bilaterally on the pelvic limb upon palpation.
- **Nervous system**: Normal – BAR. CNs intact. Facial sensation intact with no evidence of facial asymmetry. Full neuro exam not performed.

Diagnostic Tests, Radiology/CT Report

- Mild to moderate, bilateral, stifle osteoarthrosis with mild to moderate intracapsular swelling (L>R).
- Conclusion: Pelvic limb lameness is attributed to the lesions in the stifles; the radiographic findings are consistent with the clinical diagnosis of cranial cruciate ligament injury.

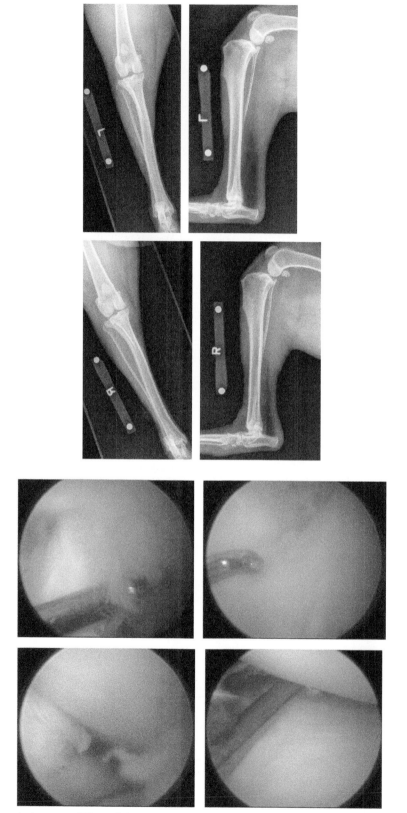

Arthroscopy: CCL partial rupture and intact meniscus.

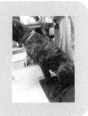

Case #3

CC: Bilateral hindlimb lameness, 3 months' duration
Age: Young (1 year 10 months old)
Size: Giant (51.8 kg), Mastiff (SF)
Problem: Bilateral CCL disease (partial, chronic) intact meniscus

History

A 1.5-year-old female spayed Mastiff presented for evaluation of lameness of both bilateral hindlimbs.

- Three months ago, she was outside running when the owner saw her fall. She got up limping and fell again. She was taken to her primary care veterinarian, who sent her home with meloxicam.
- Approximately two weeks later she fell again when walking and when she stood up she was lame in both hindlimbs.
- The owner reports that she shows more lameness in the left hindlimb than the right.
- She is currently on carprofen 100 mg twice a day and a glucosamine supplement.

Physical Examination

- **Musculoskeletal**: Abnormal – ambulatory x4, but mildly ataxic on hindlimbs, mild bilateral hindlimb muscle atrophy, bilateral positive tibial trust and cranial drawer, moderate bilateral stifle effusion, moderate to severe bilateral medial buttress (worse on R>L), no neck or back pain, symmetric forelimb musculature, resists hip extension bilaterally (mildly painful).
- **Nervous system**: Normal – pupillary light reflex (PLR) intact bilateral, menace intact, CP x4 normal, spinal reflexes intact.

Diagnostic Tests, Radiology/CT Report

- Mild osteoarthrosis with moderate intracapsular swelling, left stifle.
- Mild to moderate osteoarthrosis with moderate intracapsular swelling and questionable OCD lesion, right stifle.
- Mild osteoarthrosis and mild to moderate joint incongruity, bilateral hip joints (R>L).
- Mild muscle atrophy, right pelvic limb.
- Congenital tibial malformations, bilateral.
- Conclusion: Lameness is attributed to the lesion in both the hips and stifles. Stifle intracapsular swelling can be due to any cause of synovitis, with ligamentous instability (CCL rupture) being most likely. The results of this evaluation are positive for hip dysplasia. The lucency in the right femoral condyle is only a questionable OCD lesion, as it could be artifact due to superimposed osteophytes.
- The conclusions described in this report are based on the available information. If additional images (or other information) are obtained, then these conclusions might change.

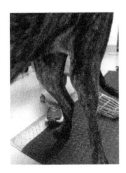

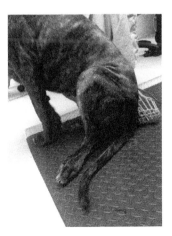

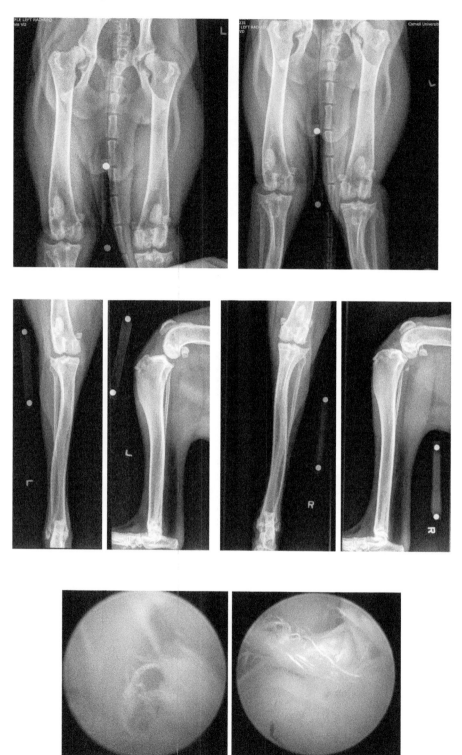

Arthroscopy: Partial CCL rupture, no OCD.

Case #4

CC: Bilateral hindlimb lameness; left: chronic, right: acute
Age: Mature (10 years old)
Size: Large (34.7 kg), Golden Retriever mix (SF)
Problem: Bilateral CCL disease (complete, chronic), meniscal injury

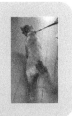

Video 11.2 Pelvic limb lameness, worse on the right (CCLD).

History

A 10-year-old spayed female Golden Retriever who presented for bilateral hindlimb lameness. She lives an active life and appears generally systemically healthy.

- She had a history of mild lameness after activity on her left pelvic limb until six months ago, when she became acutely lame and non-weight bearing on the limb.
- She was medically managed by her primary veterinarian with meloxicam and Phycox once daily, and has used a brace for this leg as well. She is also assisted with a harness while walking.
- She has been compensating well until last week when she became acutely lame on her right pelvic limb. She returned to her primary veterinarian and was prescribed 75 mg tramadol twice daily in addition to her current pain control regimen.
- She is otherwise healthy and no vomiting, diarrhea, coughing, sneezing, or changes in her eating/drinking/urinating/defecating behaviors were reported.

Physical Examination

- **Musculoskeletal**: Abnormal – severe toe-touching lameness of right hindlimb. Severe bilateral stifle instability when walked. Bilateral drawer and thrust, effusion appreciated.

Pain on manipulation of both stifles. Right clinically worse compared to left.

- **Nervous system**: Normal – incomplete neuro exam, but only deficit appreciated was slow paw placement of right hindlimb, but this was attributed to toe-touching lameness.

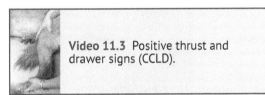

Video 11.3 Positive thrust and drawer signs (CCLD).

Diagnostic Tests, Radiology/CT Report

- Left crus: Within the stifle joint, a moderate increased soft tissue opacity displaces the infrapatellar fat pad cranially and the gastrocnemius fascia caudally. Along the periarticular margins of the patella, femoral trochlear ridges, and femoral and tibial condyles, small osteophytes are detected.
- Right crus: Within the stifle joint, mild to moderate increased soft tissue opacity displaces the infrapatellar fat pad cranially and the gastrocnemius fascia caudally. Minimal osteophytes are suspected at the distal patella.
- Summary:
  - Moderate intracapsular swelling with mild osteoarthrosis, left stifle.
  - Mild to moderate intracapsular swelling with minimal osteoarthrosis, right stifle.
- Conclusion: Lameness can be attributed to the cause of bilateral stifle joint swelling and osteoarthrosis, with a primary differential diagnosis of ligament instability (e.g., cranial cruciate ligament rupture).

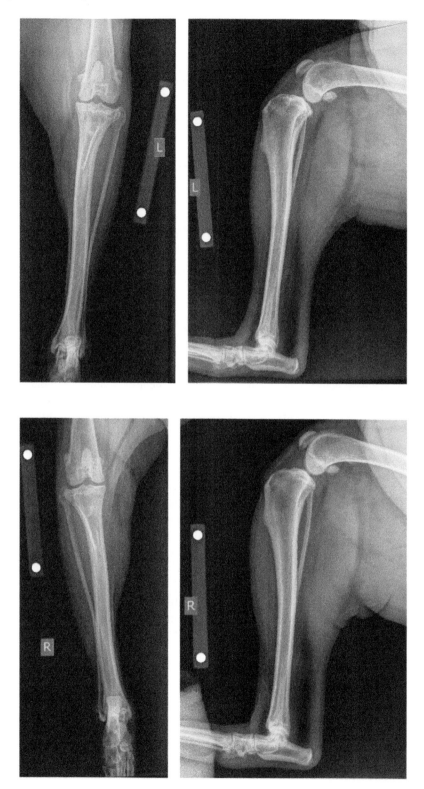

11.2 Cruciate Disease and Medial Patellar Luxation

> **Case #5**
>
> **CC**: Bilateral hindlimb lameness
> **Age**: Mature (5 years 9 months old)
> **Size**: Small (4.4 kg), Yorkshire Terrier (MN)
> **Problem**: CCL disease and medial patellar luxation (MPL, grade 3) (confirmed), hip osteoarthritis

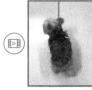

> Video 11.4 Pelvic limb gait abnormality (MPL and CCLD).

History

A male castrated Yorkshire Terrier, 5 years and 9 months old, presented for right hindlimb lameness for a few months and left hindlimb lameness for four weeks.

- He was previously diagnosed with bilateral patellar luxation

Physical Examination

- **Musculoskeletal**: Abnormal – bilateral luxated patellas (grade 3/4), positive drawer and tibial thrust left stifle, mildly lame left hindlimb, sits with left leg rotated laterally.
- **Nervous system**: Normal – normal menace, palpebral, normal conscious proprioception.

Diagnostic Tests, Radiology/CT Report

- Bilateral medial patellar luxation with crural malformation.
- Mild intracapsular effusion, cranial tibial subluxation, and mild osteoarthrosis, left stifle (CCL rupture).
- Right hip dysplasia with moderate osteoarthrosis.

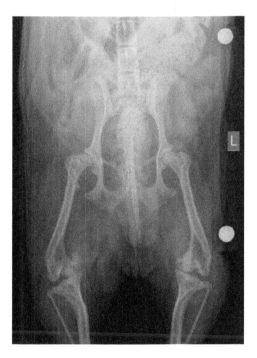

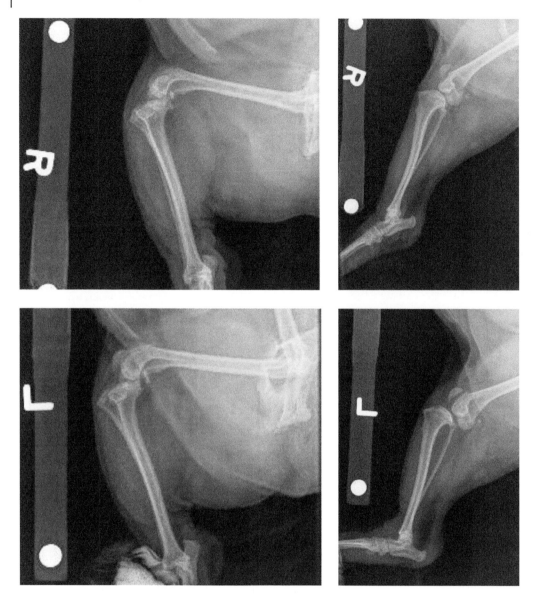

Case #6

CC: Right hindlimb lameness
Age: Mature (3 years old)
Size: Large (25.8 kg), Pitbull Terrier (SF)
Problem: CCL disease (suspect) and MPL (grade 3)

Video 11.5 Pelvic limb lameness (MPL and CCLD).

History

A 3-year-old female spayed Pitbull presented for evaluation of a 2–3-month history of right hindlimb lameness.

- Her owner reports that he first noticed her as slow to rise following long periods of rest a few months ago. He believes she has progressively become more lame and is now hardly using the leg.
- She was seen by a pet hospital and diagnosed with a medially luxating patella.
- She is an otherwise healthy dog and has had no episodes of vomiting, diarrhea, coughing, sneezing, lethargy, or inappetence, with no changes in urination or defecation. She is up to date on vaccinations and is currently not on any medications.

Physical Examination

- **Musculoskeletal**: Abnormal – three-legged lame (right hind), grade 3 medial luxating patella, evidence of muscle atrophy on right hindlimb.
- **Nervous system**: Normal – cranial nerve intact, no proprioceptive deficits noted.

Diagnostic Tests, Radiology/CT Report

- Right crus: The stifle joint has a moderate amount of increased fluid opacity that distends the joint capsule cranially and caudally, and small osteophytes on the medial femoral condyle, the lateral tibial condyle, the medial fabella, the apex of the patella, and the cranial aspect of the tibial plateau. The patella is moderately medially displaced.
- Conclusion:
  - Moderate, grade 3 patella luxation, right stifle.
  - Moderate osteoarthrosis, right stifle.

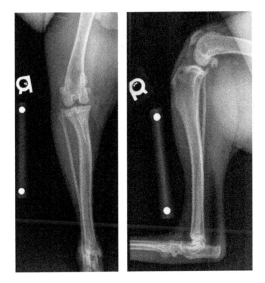

11.3   Hip Osteoarthritis

> **Case #7**
>
> **CC**: Chronic bilateral hindlimb lameness
> **Age**: Mature (3 years 6 months old)
> **Size**: Large (52.3 kg), German Shepherd (SF)
> **Problem**: Hip osteoarthritis

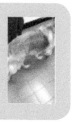

Video 11.6 Pelvic limb lameness (hip OA).

History

A 3.5-year-old female spayed German Shepherd presented for a 5–6-month history of bilateral hindlimb lameness.

- He had been previously seen by the primary care veterinarian, who suspected bilateral hip dysplasia, with shallow joint surfaces in the hip and coxofemoral joint incongruity. There were also severe osteoarthritic changes in the left hip, mild osteoarthritic changes in the right hip, and mild osteoarthritic changes in the lumbosacral space.
- Since the visit with the primary care veterinarian, the lameness has not progressed in severity. The patient is not as active as the other pets in the house and she is often more lame upon return from playing outside; she has a "bunny hop" gait after strenuous exercise.
- A one-week course of Rimadyl, prescribed by the primary care veterinarian, dramatically improved her clinical signs.

Physical Examination

- **Musculoskeletal**: Abnormal – gait: walks with a sway and bilateral hindlimb lameness, bunny hop on pivot, low back carriage, narrow-based stance in hindlimbs, pain on tail extension. Recumbent: there is crepitus in the left and right hips, which is more severe in the left hind. There is more paw-pad wear on the right hind. Normal sit test. No other abnormalities detected.

Diagnostic Tests, Radiology/CT Report

- Bilateral hip dysplasia with severe osteoarthritis (L>R).

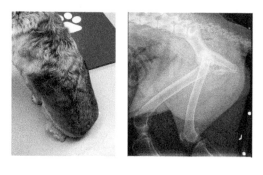

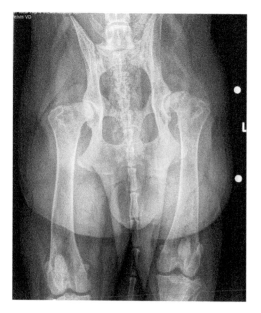

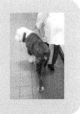

Case #8

CC: Chronic bilateral hindlimb lameness
Age: Mature (onset at six months old, presented at 11 years old)
Size: Large (39.3 kg), Old English Sheepdog (NM)
Problem: Hip osteoarthritis

Video 11.7 Pelvic limb lameness (hip OA).

History

An 11-year-old male castrated Old English Sheepdog presented for evaluation of an acute episode on chronic left hindlimb lameness.

- He was diagnosed with bilateral hip dysplasia many years ago through his primary care veterinarian.
- He has historically had bilateral hindlimb lameness, more significant on the left, since he was 6 months old. The lameness has been described as intermittent.
- He receives fish oil supplement and Dasuquin joint supplements.

Physical Examination

- **Musculoskeletal**: Abnormal – persistent bilateral hindlimb lameness; ambulation: shortened stride in both L and R hind, visible atrophy of musculature on L and R hind, holds hips internally rotated when walks. Standing exam: bears more weight on R than L hindlimb, no long bone pain, no spinal or neck pain on palpation, easily flexes and extends neck, no joint effusion, laxity, or medial buttress of stifle; no tibial thrust, cranial drawer, or crepitation palpated in stifles in lateral exam; no patellar luxation (unsedated). Pain elicited during hip extension and abduction, with the left being more severely affected. Crepitus detected in left hip with accompanying periarticular swelling.
- **Nervous system**: Normal – good proprioception, normal menace and palpebral reflexes; full neuro exam not completed.

Diagnostic Tests, Radiology/CT Report

- Moderate to severe osteoarthrosis, bilateral hip joints (L>R).
- Mild to moderate muscle atrophy, bilateral pelvic limbs (L>R).

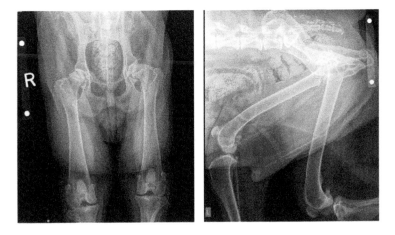

11.4 Lumbosacral Disease

> **Case #9**
>
> **CC**: Chronic bilateral hindlimb ataxia
> **Age**: Mature (10 years old)
> **Size**: Large (40 kg), German Shepherd (NM)
> **Problem**: Lumbosacral disease

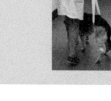

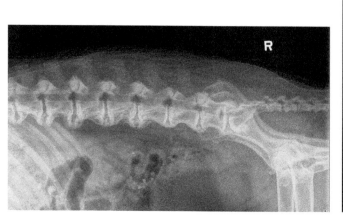

Video 11.8 Pelvic limb ataxia (LS disease).

History

A 10-year-old male castrated German Shepherd presented for exercise intolerance. A 4DX snap test was also performed and was negative.

- Two years ago, he was diagnosed with Lyme and *Anaplasma phagocytophilum*. He is up to date on all vaccinations except for kennel cough. He is on a flea and tick preventative.

Physical Examination

- **Musculoskeletal**: Abnormal – ambulatory x4, no pain on long bone palpation, no joint swelling, normal symmetric musculature; full ortho exam not performed, moderate muscle atrophy of caudal thighs and epaxials.
- **Nervous system**: Abnormal – mild generalized proprioceptive ataxia (on opioids at time of exam), urine dribbling, CN reflexes intact, normal paw placement x4, no pain on spinal palpation, resented lifting of the tail.

Diagnostic Tests, Radiology/CT Report

- Lumbosacral spondylosis deformans with mild articular process osteoarthrosis.
- Incompletely characterized hip osteoarthrosis.
- The results of this evaluation are negative for an aggressive bone lesion. A cause for the clinical signs is not determined.

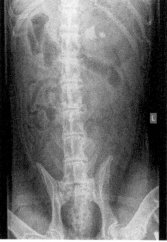

11.5   Hip Luxation

Case #10

CC: Trauma, acute left hindlimb lameness
Age: Mature (3 years 6 months old)
Size: Small (9.9 kg), Cocker Spaniel (F)
Problem: Craniodorsal hip luxation

Video 11.9a Pelvic limb lameness (hip luxation).

Video 11.9b Pelvic limb lameness (view from side) (hip luxation).

History

A 3-year-old female intact Cocker Spaniel presented for evaluation and care following a motor vehicle accident.

- She was hit by a car traveling at approximately 30 miles per hour. The incident was not directly observed. Immediately afterward, she was found recumbent in the road and unable or unwilling to walk.
- She was immediately brought to her primary care veterinarian, who gave subcutaneous fluids. During this visit, she was reportedly observed to walk. Her owners feel she is very quiet since being hit by the car.
- She is otherwise healthy and not on any medications.

Physical Examination

- **Musculoskeletal**: Abnormal – dorsal deviation of left greater trochanter, forming a straight line with the ischiatic tuberosity and iliac crest. Painful on palpation of the left greater trochanteric region. Nonpainful boney palpation otherwise, and stable joints otherwise (with the exception of the left coxofemoral joint as described above).
- **Nervous system**: Abnormal – mentation: dull though responsive. Cranial nerves: see strabismus above, otherwise normal. Spinal reflexes: withdrawal x4 within normal limits (WNL) (sluggish left rear though present), patellar reflexes x2 WNL. Proprioception: delayed CP left forelimb though possibly due to discomfort from the intra-venous catheter (IVC), not performed on left rear as patient would not allow extension of the limb. Normal hopping on all limbs other than left rear. Patient is ambulatory, though non-weight bearing on the left rear.

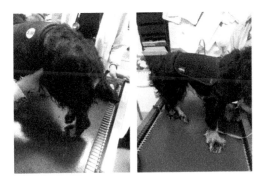

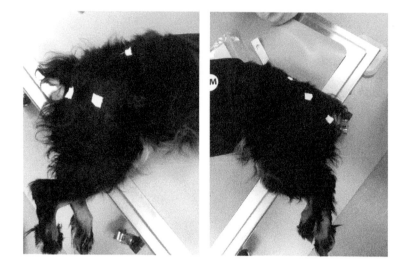

Diagnostic Tests, Radiology/CT Report

- Craniodorsal hip luxation, left.
- Conclusion: The results of this evaluation confirm reluxation of the left hip joint.

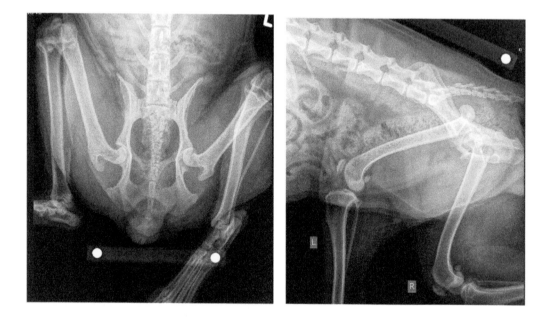

11.6   Calcaneal Tendon Pathology

Case #11

CC: Left pelvic limb lameness
Age: Mature (7 years old)
Size: Large (41.4 kg), Labrador Retriever (SF)
Problem: Calcaneal tendon complete rupture

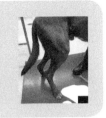

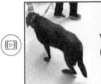

Video 11.10 Pelvic limb lameness (calcaneal tendon rupture).

History

A 7-year-old, female spayed, chocolate Labrador Retriever was referred for laceration of her left gastrocnemius tendon.

- Earlier that day, she ran in front of her owner, who was cross-country skiing, and they got into an accident. Her left hock was cut and bleeding, and she was only able to bear weight on three limbs. Her owners were able to bandage the bleeding within 15 minutes of the accident and brought her to her primary care veterinarian immediately. It was determined that there was a full laceration of the left gastrocnemius tendon, and she was referred.
- Otherwise she has been relatively healthy. She does have osteoarthritis of her left and right stifles and hips; she is given Deramaxx, fish oil, and chondroitin/glucosamine to control her symptoms. She is up to date on vaccines and has a Seresto collar for flea and tick control.

Physical Examination

- **Musculoskeletal**: Abnormal – weight bearing x3. Plantigrade stance of left hindlimb. Laceration of the L gastrocnemius tendon.

No damage to bones or hock joint noted. No fractures palpated. Pain with decreased range of movement of stifles and hips bilaterally.

- **Nervous system**: Normal.

Diagnostic Tests, Radiology/CT Report

- The soft tissues in the plantarodistal crus are thick and contain a linear laceration through the common calcaneal tendon approximately 1.5 cm proximal to the calcaneal tubercle. Bone or joint involvement is not detected.
- Conclusion: Acute, traumatic, left common calcaneal tendon laceration.

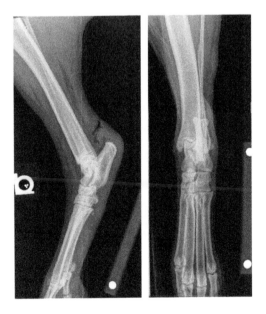

Case #12

CC: Left pelvic limb lameness
Age: Mature (4 years old)
Size: Medium (18.2 kg), Whippet (NM)
Problem: Calcaneal (gastrocnemius) tendon rupture with intact superficial digital flexor

Video 11.11 Pelvic limb lameness (gastrocnemius tendon rupture).

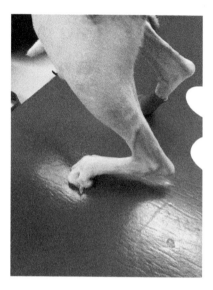

History

A 4.5-year-old male castrated Whippet presented for left hindlimb lameness.

- Five months ago, he dislocated a toe on his right hind leg while chasing a squirrel. After the injury, he was walking abnormally on his right hind foot and subsequently developed a wound on the lateral aspect.
- Three months ago, he was diagnosed with left Achilles' tendon degeneration and has subsequently been treated with braces.

Physical Examination

- **Musculoskeletal**: Abnormal – left dropped hock, "crab-claw," decreased weight-bearing due to left calcaneal tendon rupture; R toes divert to the left due to ligamentous injury.
- **Nervous system**: Normal – CN reflexes intact, no evidence of ataxia; full neuro exam not performed.

Diagnostic Tests, Ultrasonography/CT Report

- Previous left gastrocnemius rupture.
- Progressive severe diffuse left gastrocnemius tendinopathy.
- Probable locally extensive adhesion, left gastrocnemius to superficial digital flexor.
- Uncertain status, left conjoined tendinopathy.

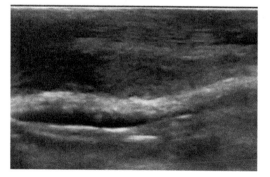

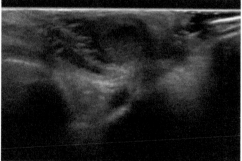

11.7 Neoplasia

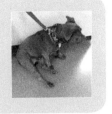

Case #13

CC: Right pelvic limb lameness
Age: Mature (7 years old)
Size: Medium (26.3 kg), Pitbull mix (SF)
Problem: Stifle neoplasia (suspect)

History

An 8-year-old female spayed American Staffordshire Terrier presented for lethargy and right hindlimb pain.

- She was diagnosed with chronic kidney disease and hypothyroidism, as well as right hydronephrosis and hydroureter.
- She has a previous history of hypothyroidism, monocortical fracture of the left ulna, and facial paralysis.

Physical Examination

- **Musculoskeletal**: Abnormal – right femoral distal long bone pain, right tibial proximal and distal long bone pain, possibly referred pain from femur, left tibial long bone pain.
- **Nervous system**: Abnormal – facial paralysis; delayed palpebral reflex both eyes (OU);

normal hopping and placement in all limbs; no pain on head/cervical/spinal palpation; normal withdrawal/popliteal reflexes.

Diagnostic Tests, Radiology/CT Report

- Probable moderate enthesopathy, right cranial and caudal cruciate ligaments.
- A definitive cause for the lameness is not determined during this evaluation.
- The enthesopathy is likely chronic and incidental because of the lack of intracapsular swelling.
- Erosive monoarthropathy and polyostotic aggressive bone lesion associated with synovial mass, right stifle.
- Right pelvic lameness is attributed to this finding, for which primary differential diagnosis is synovial neoplasia (e.g., histiocytic sarcoma, synovial cell sarcoma, metastasis, etc.).

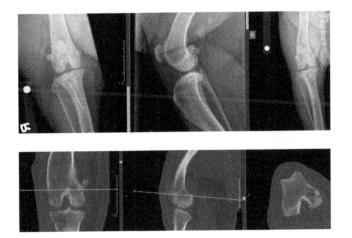

Case #14

CC: Right pelvic limb lameness
Age: Mature (9 years old)
Size: Large (23.1 kg), Pitbull mix (SF)
Problem: Primary bone tumor (probable osteosarcoma)

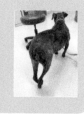

Video 11.12a Pelvic limb lameness (neoplasia).

Video 11.12b Pelvic limb lameness at trot (neoplasia).

History

A 9-year-old female spayed Pitbull mix presented for further evaluation of non-weight-bearing lameness in her right hindlimb.

- Approximately one month ago, she started limping on her right hindlimb. However, the lameness resolved within a few days.
- Approximately three weeks ago, she became non-weight bearing on her right hindlimb. Her owner administered aspirin (325 mg once to twice daily), which seemed to make her more comfortable. She has not received aspirin since.
- She has a history of dilated cardiomyopathy, which has a presumptive nutritional etiology. Her heart disease is currently well controlled with enalapril and pimobendan, and her systolic function has continued to improve.
- Her appetite has been slightly decreased for the past several days, and she has been waking up in the middle of the night crying in pain.
- Her owner does not report any recent vomiting, diarrhea, or coughing.

Physical Examination

- **Musculoskeletal**: Abnormal – moderate atrophy of the right thigh muscles. Pain on extension of the right hip. No pain on long bone palpation.
- **Nervous system**: Normal – normal menace response and palpebral reflexes. Normal mentation. Normal withdrawal reflexes. Full neurologic exam not performed.

Diagnostic Tests, Radiology/CT Report

- Monostotic, aggressive bone lesion of the right femoral diaphysis.
- The primary differential diagnosis is a primary bone tumor (osteosarcoma, fibrosarcoma, chondrosarcoma), lymphoma, less likely metastatic disease or fungal osteomyelitis.
- Spondylosis deformans, L3–L4, L5–L6, L7–S1.

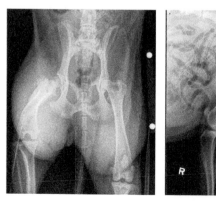

11.8   Immune-Mediated Poly-arthropathy, Septic Arthritis

> ### Case #15
>
> **CC**: Bilateral hindlimb lameness
> **Age**: Mature (6 years old)
> **Size**: Small (7.8 kg), Lhasa Apso (F)
> **Problem**: Immune-mediated poly-arthropathy (IMPA), erosive

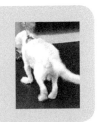

Video 11.13 Pelvic limb gait abnormality (IMPA).

History

A 6-year-old female intact Lhasa Apso presented for evaluation of suspected bilateral CCL disease – presumptively diagnosed by the Neurology Service after presenting for difficulty using her hindlimbs.

- 3–4 months ago, she began having trouble getting up from lying down.
- The problem has become progressively worse over time, with her right hindlimb more severely affected than her left.
- She has been taken to her primary care veterinarian for the issue, who performed a steroid trial, but she did not improve with steroid administration and was tapered off about a month ago.
- Recently, she has not been able to stand without help. Once she is stood up, she is able to walk with short steps in her hindlimbs. Her owners have noticed progressive muscle atrophy (right hind worse than left).
- She has been urinating, defecating, eating, and drinking normally.
- She is not up to date on her vaccines due to having a fever at her last vaccination appointment about one month ago, which resolved

without treatment. She does not receive flea/tick/heartworm preventatives. Her last heat was about three weeks ago. She is currently on carprofen (2.2 mg/kg) and pregabalin (2 mg/kg – for control of neuropathic pain) as prescribed.

Physical Examination

- **Musculoskeletal**: Abnormal – severe lameness in hindlimbs; bilaterally enlarged stifles on palpation; decreased range of motion in elbows and stifles. Pain elicited when attempting cranial drawer test in both hindlimbs. Diffuse moderate muscle atrophy in both hindlimbs (R>L). Pain on palpation of caudal cervical region.
- **Nervous system**: Normal – appropriate mentation; CN intact bilaterally; PLR and menace intact bilaterally; palpebral reflexes (medial and lateral) intact bilaterally; abnormal gait: nonambulatory paraparetic when down. If helped up on hindlimbs, she is able to walk with short steps – likely secondary to orthopedic disease; full neuro exam not performed.

Diagnostic Tests, Radiology/CT Report

- Severe, chronic erosive poly-arthropathy, left and right tarsi, left and right stifles and interphalangeal joints. The changes in all the joints are consistent with the erosive poly-arthropathy, with idiopathic vs. rheumatoid (immune-mediated) causes the most likely diagnosis.

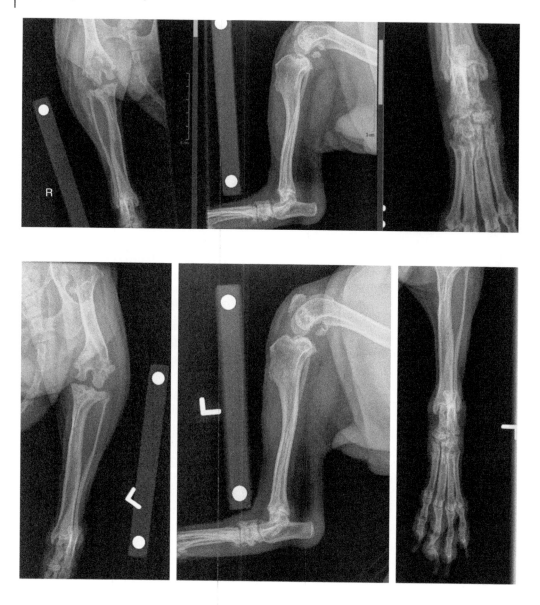

Case #16

CC: Right non-weight bearing hindlimb lameness, right hindlimb swelling
Age: Mature (4 years old)
Size: Giant (54.0 kg), Newfoundland mix (MN)
Problem: Chronic hip osteoarthritis, septic arthritis (*Staphylococcus pseudintermedius*)

Video 11.14 Pelvic limb lameness (septic arthritis).

History

A 4-year-old male castrated mixed-breed dog presented for a three-day history of lethargy, pain, and right hindlimb edema.

- He has historical bilateral hip dysplasia.
- About seven months ago, he initially became severely lame after an incident with another dog.
- About a month ago, a presumptive bacterial infection of his right hip joint (septic arthritis) was treated with cephalexin.
- About three days ago, he began to act more lethargically and was limping more than usual.
- Two days ago, his owners noticed pitting edema on his right hindlimb, and he was presented to an emergency clinic. He was prescribed cephalexin, an antibiotic, for a recurrence of the possible bacterial osteomyelitis. Chest radiographs performed at that time were reported to be free of metastatic disease. Blood work was largely unremarkable other than suspected toxic neutrophil changes and bands.
- He was presented to another emergency service for further evaluation due to apparent worsening in terms of pain, lethargy, pitting edema, and hyporexia.
- He has had no coughing, sneezing, vomiting, constipation, melena, or hematochezia.
- He has had skin infections intermittently his whole life. He is not polyuric, polyphagic, or polydipsic.

- He is currently receiving gabapentin at 300 mg every 12–24 hours, meloxicam at 7.5 mg every 24 hours, cephalexin at 1500 mg every 12 hours, and Cosequin.

Physical Examination

- **Musculoskeletal**: Abnormal – narrow-based stance. Painful on manipulation of hips and hindlimbs. Severe crepitus palpated in hips. Decreased weight bearing on right hindlimb. Offloading weight onto front limbs.
- **Full ortho exam findings**: Limited range of motion (ROM) on right hindlimb (physically difficult to manipulate, marked pain response). Right stifle edematous but suspect effusion. Left stifle stable, no cranial drawer or tibial thrust appreciated on sedated exam, no joint effusion appreciated. Crepitus and limited ROM in left hind hip. Can rise and sit on own. Offloading onto forelimbs at a sit.
- **Neurological**: Normal – normal mentation. Cranial nerves within normal limits. Full neuro exam not performed.

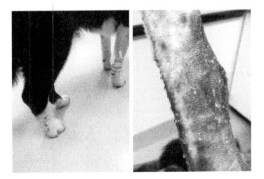

Diagnostic Tests, Radiology/CT Report

- Multifocal, large, right pelvic limb abscessations with severe, diffuse cellulitis/fasciitis.
- Severe, locally extensive, erosive monoarthropathy with osteomyelitis, right hip joint.
- Multifocal, mild to severe lymphadenopathy, right medial iliac, right internal iliac, right inguinal lymph nodes.
- Bilateral, severe right and left hip dysplasia with osteoarthrosis.
- Incidental spondylosis deformans, L5, L6.
- Likely incidental vacuum phenomenon, left hip joint.
- Acute onset of right pelvic limb lameness is attributed to the first finding. The seeding source of the infection is most likely attributed to chronic right hip septic arthritis. Lymphadenopathy is consistent with inflammatory reaction.

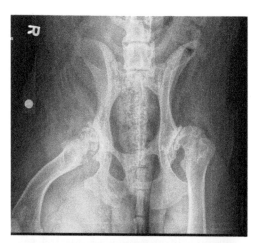

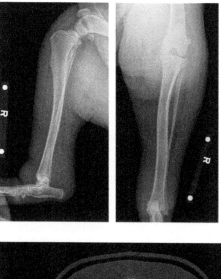

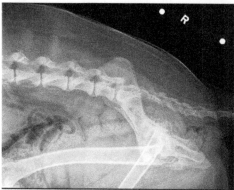

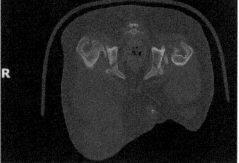

Aerobic/anaerobic culture results: *Staphylococcus pseudintermedius*

The videos are available for this chapter on www.wiley.com/go/hayashi/lameness.

12

Multiple Limb Lameness

12.1 Poly-arthropathy

Case #1

Chief Complaint (CC): Shifting limb lameness and multiple joint swelling
Age: Young (10 months old)
Size: Large (28.6 kg), German Shepherd (NM)
Problem: Immune-mediated poly-arthropathy (IMPA) (idiopathic)

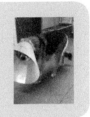

Video 12.1 Gait abnormality (IMPA).

History

A 10-month-old male castrated German Shepherd presented for evaluation of worsening of prednisone-responsive, effusive intermittent, shifting leg lameness.

- About two months ago, he developed a shifting leg lameness.
- He was 4DX negative and radiographs were not performed. Panosteitis and a urinary tract infection were suspected. He was started on prednisone (owner believes 20 mg orally twice a day) and an antibiotic (possible doxycycline). He improved, but continued to be mildly intermittently lame.

- About two weeks later, he was having a hard time getting up and radiographs of his hips were taken. They appeared normal according to the owner. A prednisone taper was attempted and he became worse again.
- He was seen again four days later, when he was started on gabapentin, amoxicillin, and ciprofloxacin, and the prednisone was increased back to the original dose. He improved and his prednisone was tapered again. He was completely off of prednisone for two weeks about a month ago, from when he has been mildly lame and had a decreased appetite, but was otherwise doing ok.
- About a week ago, he worsened again and was seen at the referring veterinarian for hyporexia and lameness. Cerenia was prescribed as well as gabapentin, amoxicillin, ciprofloxacin, and prednisone. The antibiotics were prescribed for one week. He has been febrile at each referring veterinarian

visit for about three months; the owner reports a temperature of 106.8 °F as well as a leukocytosis.

- He improved with these medications and prednisone taper was started. He received 20 mg twice a day, 10 mg twice a day, and 10 mg once a day last week.

- Since yesterday, he has been toe-touching lame on his left front limb and hyporexic again. The owner gave an additional 10 mg of prednisone prior to presentation today.

- Current medications prednisone 10 mg orally once a day (0.35 mg/kg/day), gabapentin 600 mg orally q8–12h.

- He has otherwise been healthy, with no diarrhea or vomiting for about three months. Owner does take him on wooded hikes and runs. He swims in lakes and creeks. Never found any ticks on him.

Physical Examination

- Temp 104.3 °F.
- **Musculoskeletal**: ambulatory x4 with moderate left forelimb lameness; mild elbow effusion (L>R), and discomfort to palpation/extension of left. Mild to moderate bilateral tarsal effusion and warmth. No discomfort on long bone palpation. Complete orthopedic examination not performed
- **Neurologic**: no neurologic deficits/abnormalities on brief exam.

Diagnostic Tests, Radiology/Computed Tomography (CT) Report

- Mild intracapsular swelling, left elbow.
- Impression: The lameness is likely attributed to the cause of the intracapsular swelling (presumed effusion), the underlying cause for which is not determined in this evaluation.

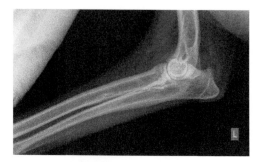

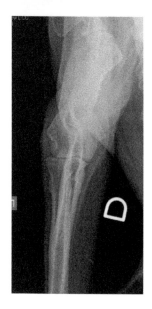

- Thoracic radiographs: negative for thoracic metastasis.

Other Diagnostic Tests

- Abdominal ultrasound: mild diffuse hepatopathy; mild cholestasis.
- C-reactive protein (CRP): 29.9 mg/L (0.0–12.0).
- Urine culture: no growth.
- Joint fluid cytology: marked neutrophilic inflammation in multiple joints, consistent with IMPA.

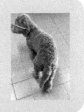

Case #2

CC: Bilateral thoracic limb lameness and left pelvic limb lameness
Age: Young (7 months old)
Size: Medium (15.2 kg at 7 months), Labradoodle (F)
Problem: Lyme disease (suspected)

Video 12.2a Pelvic limb lameness (Lyme disease).

Video 12.2b Thoracic limb lameness (Lyme disease).

History

A 6-month-old female intact Labradoodle presented for an evaluation of acute onset of lameness.

- The owner reported lameness in both of the front legs and left hindlimb, and discomfort on palpation of both forelimbs (particularly elbows), right hind foot, and both hips. She has had trouble rising from a lying position. She has been quieter for three days and no injuries were seen.
- She still has normal appetite and no vomiting, diarrhea, coughing, or sneezing. She is not on any medications currently and is up to date on vaccinations.

Physical Examination

- **Musculoskeletal**: Abnormal – ambulatory x4 with left hindlimb lameness.
  - Spinal palpation: no pain elicited on paraspinal palpation; normal neck range of movement (ROM) with no pain elicited.
  - Gait: mild weight-bearing grade 1/4 left hindlimb lameness, most evident at a trot.
  - Standing: after orthopedic exam, is toe-touching on left hindlimb when standing.
  - Sit test: holds limbs out to the side when sitting (equal preference for left and right).
  - Right thoracic limb: decreased flexion in carpus, moderate increased medial and lateral carpus laxity, noticeable valgus of the antebrachium, shortened antebrachium, no elbow or carpal effusion, no long bone pain, normal ROM in shoulder and manus.
  - Left thoracic limb: decreased extension in carpus, moderate increased medial and lateral carpus laxity, noticeable valgus of the antebrachium, shortened antebrachium, no elbow or carpal effusion, no long bone pain, normal ROM in shoulder and manus.
  - Pelvic limbs: mild to moderate stifle effusion bilaterally (left worse than right), femur pain on palpation bilaterally, pain on stifle and hip extension bilaterally. No instability or altered ROM identified; no cranial drawer or tibial thrust elicited bilaterally.

Diagnostic Tests

- SNAP 4Dx test Lyme positive.

Medications Prescribed

- Doxycycline 150 mg (10 mg/kg) orally once a day for 28 days.
- Gabapentin 100 mg (6.5 mg/kg) orally two to three times a day as needed.
- Meloxicam (1.5 mg/mL oral suspension): 1 mL (0.1 mg/kg) orally once a day, to give if persistent pain after 2–3 days of doxycycline treatment.

Plan

- If she is still painful and/or lame after 2–3 days of treatment for Lyme, treat for suspected panosteitis.

12.2   Bilateral Stifle Osteochondritis Dissecans and Cruciate Disease

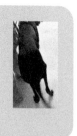

Case #3

CC: Chronic bilateral hindlimb lameness
Age: Young (1 year old)
Size: Giant (55.5 kg), Great Dane (M)
Problem: Bilateral stifle osteochondritis dissecans (OCD), septic arthritis (iatrogenic), and cranial cruciate ligament (CCL) disease

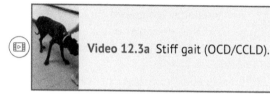

Video 12.3a Stiff gait (OCD/CCLD).

Video 12.3b Pelvic limb lameness (OCD/CCLD).

History

A 1-year-old intact male Great Dane presented for an 11-month history of bilateral hindlimb lameness (R>>L), which has continued and worsened after diagnosis of bilateral OCD and surgery performed 10 months ago.

- Current medications: carprofen 125 mg twice a day (last given last night), helping, increased recently.
- At 6 months of age, he came home with sudden lameness from doggy daycare. Diagnosed with bilateral OCD. Received open-stifle surgery bilaterally and developed multiple drug resistance (MDR). He was doing okay for a while, then R stifle flared up and was flushed two more times, which also helped. He would get better, but then days to weeks after coming off antibiotics would develop lameness again.

Lameness most improved on Simplicef (prescribed for puppy dermatitis) and lameness started again a few days after antibiotics course ended so it was restarted and finished two months ago.

- Exercise worsens lameness. He is at his normal baseline lameness right now.

Physical Examination

- **Musculoskeletal**: Abnormal – ambulatory x4 with grade 3/5 right hindlimb lameness. Bilateral stifle effusion and crepitus (R>L). Reduced range of motion of R stifle. Severe diffuse muscle atrophy of right hindlimb. No instability – no cranial drawer or tibial thrust bilaterally.
- **Nervous system:** Normal mentation. No apparent paresis or ataxia. Normal menace, palpebral reflex intact, normal pupillary light reflex present in both eyes (OU).

Diagnostic Tests, Radiology/CT Report

- Severe erosive arthropathy with moderate intracapsular effusion, right stifle.
- Moderate erosive arthropathy with moderate intracapsular effusion and two intraarticular mineral bodies, left stifle.
- Impression: Erosive arthropathy is likely associated with the previously diagnosed septic arthritis. Although septic arthritis was not reported in the left stifle, an infectious etiology is similarly possible in this limb as well. Differentiation between a

discrete OCD lesion and erosive lesions secondary to the septic arthritis is not possible; thus, while measurements are provided for the largest defect of the right stifle, it is unclear if this coincides with the location of the previously diagnosed OCD lesion or a newer, erosive lesion. Limited range of motion associated with the right stifle is primarily attributed to severe, chronic degenerative joint disease, presumed secondary to the previously diagnosed septic arthritis and OCD lesion. The intraarticular mineral bodies of the left stifle are of unclear clinical significance, and may represent joint capsule mineralization, OCD fragment(s), small avulsion fragments (of unknown etiology), or small joint mice of alternate etiology.

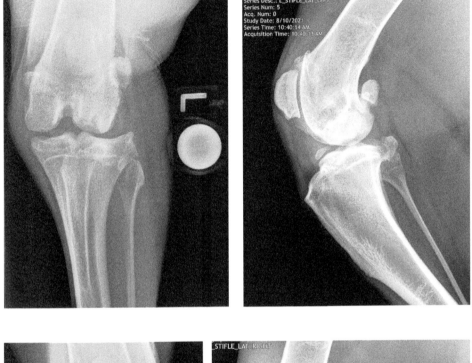

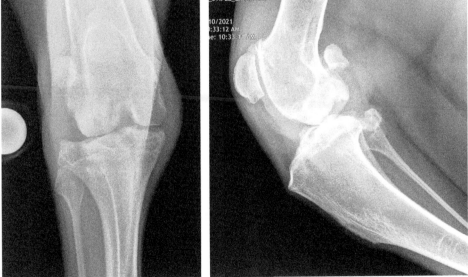

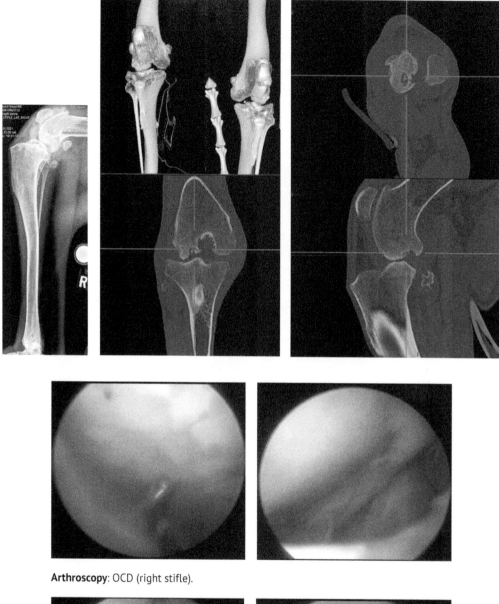

Arthroscopy: OCD (right stifle).

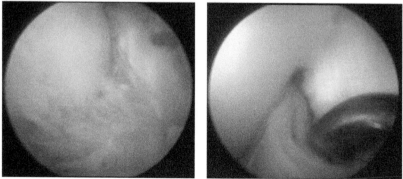

CCL partial rupture (right stifle).

12.3 Bilateral Hip Luxation, Cruciate Disease, and Medial Patellar Luxation

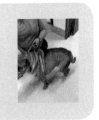

Case #4

CC: Acute left hindlimb lameness
Age: Mature (5 years old)
Size: Medium (20.6 kg), Sharpei (NM)
Problem: Bilateral CCL disease

Video 12.4 Non-weight bearing posture (CCLD/hip luxation).

History

A 5-year-old male neutered Chinese Sharpei presenting for progressive left hindlimb lameness.

- A couple weeks ago owner noticed he was hopping on his left hind. He was given gabapentin for a couple days and he started using his foot again.
- About 1.5 weeks ago owner took him on a 20-minute walk, he would not bear weight on his left hind and was hopping. Owner took him to the vet last week, who took radiographs and diagnosed him with a torn left CCL and bilateral hip dysplasia.

Physical Examination

- **Musculoskeletal**: Non-weight bearing on left hindlimb with stifle joint instability and positive thrust. No pain on hip extension either side. Right hind grade 2/4 medial patellar luxation.

Diagnostic Tests, Radiology/CT Report

- Bilateral craniodorsal coxofemoral luxation.
- Bilateral hip dysplasia and moderate degenerative osteoarthrosis.
- Bilateral medial patellar luxation.
- Moderate intracapsular swelling and mild osteoarthrosis, left stifle and right stifle.
- Bilateral hypoplastic trochlear ridges and angular limb deformities of the femurs and tibiae.
- Mineral opaque structure medial to the left femoral head.
- Soft tissue bulge dorsal to the left metatarsal bones and thickened soft tissues plantar to the right metatarsal bones.
- Impression: Left hindlimb lameness is prioritized secondary to the cause of the left stifle joint effusion and osteoarthrosis, with CCL rupture being most likely. However, the concurrent medial patellar luxation and hip luxation on the left side may also be contributing to or causing the lameness. Bilateral hip luxation is presumed to be secondary to bilateral hip dysplasia. The right stifle joint effusion and mild osteoarthrosis may be secondary to the medial patellar luxation; however, concurrent CCL rupture (partial or complete) is

also possible. The hypoplastic trochlear ridges and angular limb deformities are likely a congenital variant. The mineral opaque structure medial to the left femoral head may be due to osteophyte formation, but a small avulsion fragment is not ruled out. The bulge and thickening of the soft tissues at the level of the metatarsal bones are likely a normal variant for the patient, but edema and cellulitis are not ruled out.

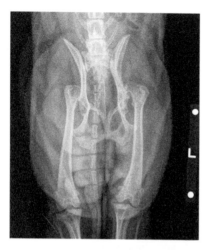

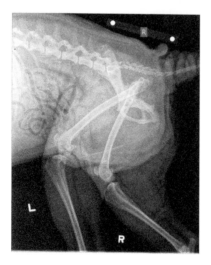

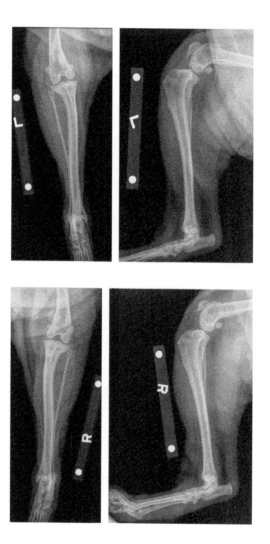

12.4 Bilateral Hip Osteoarthritis and Cruciate Disease

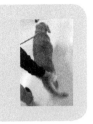

Case #5

CC: Chronic bilateral hindlimb lameness
Age: Old (12 years old)
Size: Large (33.5 kg), Golden Retriever (SF)
Problem: Bilateral hip osteoarthritis and CCL disease

Video 12.5a Pelvic limb weakness/lameness (CCLD/hip OA).

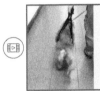

Video 12.5b Pelvic limb lameness with a sling support (CCLD/hip OA).

History

A female spayed Golden Retriever, 11 years and 7 months old, presenting for progressive hindlimb weakness.

- She began experiencing hindlimb weakness six months ago, but it has gotten worse over the past month. Initially she began having trouble going up stairs, but is now collapsing frequently on flat ground. She was given Adequan injections by the referring veterinarian, but did not show improvement and it was discontinued.
- About three weeks ago, she presented to a neurology service. She was found to have weakness in hindlimbs bilaterally, moderately thickened stifles and crepitus bilaterally, and a positive right hind tibial thrust and cranial drawer. Orthopedic disease was prioritized, but a diffuse neuromuscular disease was not ruled out.
- She has not had any episodes of coughing, sneezing, vomiting, or diarrhea and has been urinating and defecating normally. She has a history of seizures about six years ago, but has been managed on phenobarbital and has not had any since. She also has hypothyroidism, which has been managed with levothyroxine.

Physical Examination

- **Musculoskeletal**: Abnormal – hindlimb weakness/lameness. Collapses after several steps. Stifle effusion bilaterally. Right stifle positive cranial drawer and tibial thrust. Severe crepitus with pain in left hip and decreased ROM. Muscle atrophy over right shoulder. Right front limb lameness, with head bob noticed when hindlimbs supported by cart. No pain elicited on long bone palpation; no back pain noted.
- **Nervous system**: Appropriate mentation; normal menace, palpebral right eye (OD); normal conscious proprioception; no nystagmus or strabismus noted; no ataxia.

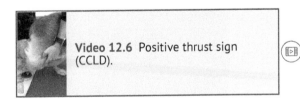

Video 12.6 Positive thrust sign (CCLD).

Diagnostic Tests, Radiology/CT Report – Thorax

- Focal moderate pulmonary venous congestion, cranial pulmonary veins.
- Mild left-sided cardiomegaly.
- Mild diffuse hepatomegaly with suspected focal hepatic mass effect.

- Impression: The focal pulmonary venous congestion and left-sided cardiomegaly may indicate early or imminent left-sided congestive heart failure, though there is no pulmonary edema detected at this time. Hepatomegaly is nonspecific, with both benign and malignant etiologies possible, and the focal displacement of the gastric lumen concerning for focal hepatic mass. The results of this evaluation are negative for thoracic metastasis.

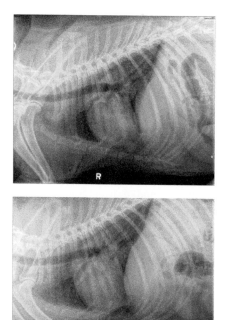

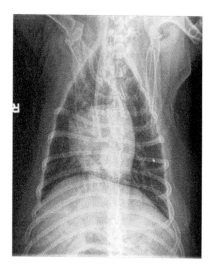

Diagnostic Tests, Radiology/CT
Report – Stifle

- Moderate right stifle osteoarthrosis, with moderate to severe intracapsular swelling and right stifle subluxation.
- Mild left stifle osteoarthrosis and intracapsular swelling.
- Moderate bilateral pelvic limb muscle atrophy.
- Moderate left tarsal osteoarthrosis.
- Small subcutaneous, fat-opaque nodule, medial aspect, left pelvic limb.
- Impression: The clinical and radiographic signs are most consistent with right CCL desmopathy. The left stifle changes are also prioritized to be secondary to cranial cruciate desmopathy (partial vs. complete tear), though other synovial injury or degenerative joint diseases are possible as well.

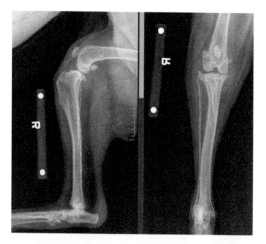

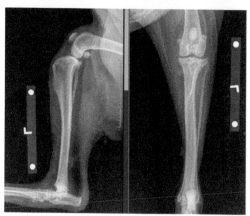

Diagnostic Tests, Radiology/CT Report – Hip

- Severe bilateral hip dysplasia and osteoarthrosis.
- Craniodorsal left hip subluxation.
- Focal mineral body craniolateral to left hip.
- Mild bilateral stifle osteoarthrosis.
- Moderate to severe bilateral pelvic limb muscle atrophy.
- Impression: Hindlimb lameness is primarily attributed to hip dysplasia and severe bilateral hip osteoarthrosis. The small mineral body craniolateral to the left hip is prioritized to be an avulsed osteophyte, though dystrophic mineralization (e.g., of the rectus femoris tendon) is possible.

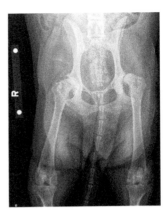

Other Diagnostic Tests

Complete blood count (CBC), blood chemistry, and urinalysis did not indicate significant systemic and oncologic conditions in this 12-year-old large-breed dog.

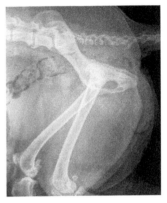

Test	Results	Unit	Lowest Value	Highest Value
HCT	40	%	41	58
HB	13.1	g/dL	14.1	20.1
RBC	5.8	mill/uL	5.7	8.5
MCV	68	fL	64	76
MCH	22	pg	21	26
MCHC	33	g/dL	33	36
RDW	13.7	%	10.6	14.3
RETICA	0.3	%	0.2	1.5
RETIC_ABS	16.9	thou/uL	11.0	92.0
NRBC	0	/100 WBC	0	1
WBC	4.4	thou/uL	5.7	14.2
SEG_NEUT	3.3	thou/uL	2.7	9.4
BAND_NEUT	0.0	thou/uL	0.0	0.1

(Continued)

Test	Results	Unit	Lowest Value	Highest Value
LYMPH	0.8	thou/uL	0.9	4.7
MONO	0.3	thou/uL	0.1	1.3
EOSIN	0.0	thou/uL	0.1	2.1
BASO	0.0	thou/uL	0.0	0.1
PLT_SMEAR	Low?			
TP REF	7.4	g/dL	5.9	7.8
PL_AP	Normal			
WBC_EX	No significant abnormalities			
RBC_MORPH	Echinocytes few			
Parasite(s)	None seen			
Hematology Comments	See PDF for results.			
Advia Interface	Advia2			
Specimen	Blood, Whole, EDTA			

Test	Results	Unit	Lowest Value	Highest Value
NA	147	mEq/L	143	150
K	4.5	mEq/L	4.1	5.4
CL	111	mEq/L	106	114
HCO3	19	mEq/L	14	24
AN GAP	22	mEq/L	17	27
NA/K	33		Not Established	
BUN	18	mg/dL	9	26
CREAT	0.6	mg/dL	0.6	1.4
CA	8.5	mg/dL	9.4	11.1
P	5.8	mg/dL	2.7	5.4
MG	1.5	mEq/L	1.5	2.1
TP	5.7	g/dL	5.5	7.2
ALB	3.5	g/dL	3.2	4.1
GLOBULIN	2.2	g/dL	1.9	3.7
A/G	1.6		0.9	1.9
GLU	77	mg/dL	68	104
ALT	50	U/L	17	95
AST	31	U/L	18	56
ALP	64	U/L	7	115
GGT	7	U/L	0	8
TBILI	0.1	mg/dL	0.0	0.2
DBILI	0.1	mg/dL	0.0	0.1

(Continued)

Test	Results	Unit	Lowest Value	Highest Value
IBILI	0.0	mg/dL	0.0	0.1
AMYL	806	U/L	322	1310
LIPASE	39	U/L	15	228
CHOL	433	mg/dL	136	392
CK	280	U/L	64	314
LDH	105	U/L	24	388
FE	185	ug/dL	97	263
TIBC	500	ug/dL	280	489
FE %SATUR	37	%	27	66
LI	8		See Comment	
HI	7		See Comment	
II	0		See Comment	
Cobas Interface	Cobas2			
Specimen	Blood, Whole, Clotted			

Test	Results	Unit	Lowest Value	Highest Value	Qualifier	Notes
VOL_UA	2.5	mL	Not Established			
COLOR_UA	Medium yellow					
TURBIDITY_UA	Clear					
SG	1.028		Not Established			
PH_DIP	7.0					
TP_DIP	100 (2+) mg/dL					
GLU_DIP	Negative					
KET_DIP	Negative					
BILI_DIP	Small					
ICTO	Positive					
BL_DIP	Negative					
WBC_SED	None seen					
RBC_SED	None seen					
BACT_SED	None seen					
EPI_SED	Very few					
SPERM_SED	None seen					
FAT_SED	Very few					
DEBRIS_SED	None Seen					
CASTS_SED	None seen					
CRYST_SED	None seen					
Specimen	Urine, Cystocentes					

The videos are available for this chapter on www.wiley.com/go/hayashi/lameness.

Index

Diagnosis of Lameness in Dogs, First Edition. Edited by Kei Hayashi.
© 2023 John Wiley & Sons, Inc. Published 2023 by John Wiley & Sons, Inc.
Companion website: www.wiley.com/go/hayashi/lameness